Made possible by funding from
Bloomberg Philanthropies

GLOBAL REPORT ON DROWNING

PREVENTING A LEADING KILLER

World Health Organization

WHO Library Cataloguing-in-Publication Data :

Global report on drowning: preventing a leading killer.

1.Drowning - prevention and control. 2.Drowning - mortality. 3.Health Policy.
4.National Health Programs. 5.Safety Management. I.World Health Organization.

ISBN 978 92 4 156478 6 (NLM classification: WA 292)

Printed in Spain.

CONTENTS

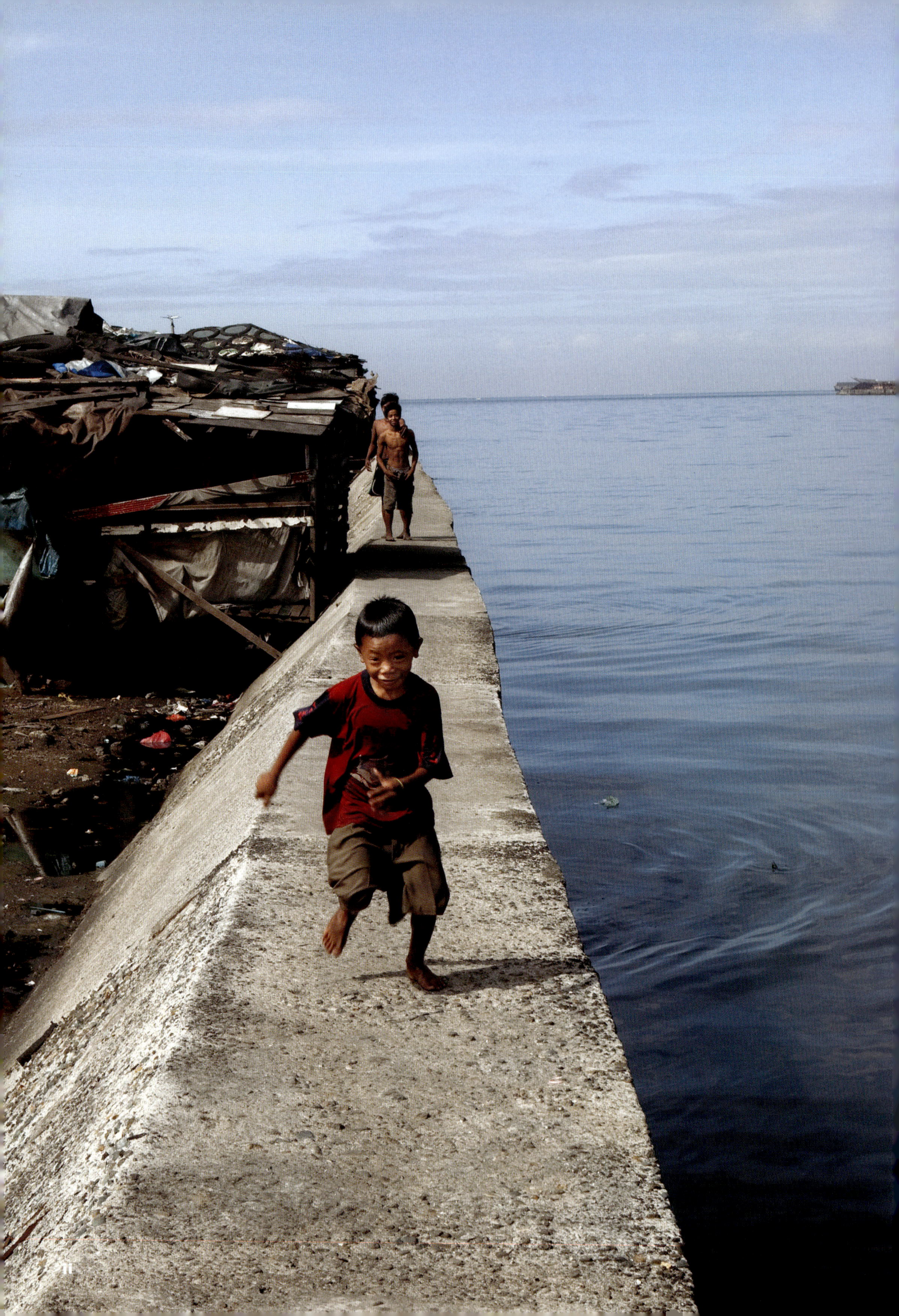

FOREWORD

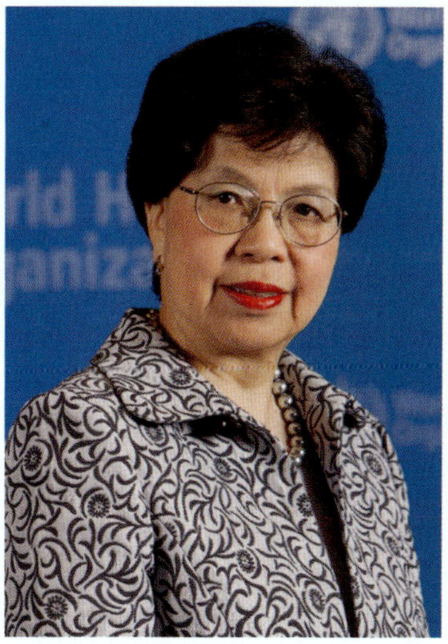

Every hour of every day more than 40 people lose their lives to drowning. Whether it is small children slipping unnoticed into a pond, pool or well; adolescents swimming under the influence of alcohol or drugs; passengers on vessels that capsize; or residents of coastal communities struck by floods, the daily toll of this leading global killer continues its quiet rise.

The Global report on drowning is the first World Health Organization report dedicated exclusively to drowning – a highly preventable public health challenge that has never been targeted by a global strategic prevention effort. This report aims to change this. It sets out current knowledge about drowning and drowning prevention, and calls for a substantial scaling up of comprehensive efforts and resources to reduce what is an intolerable death toll, particularly among children and adolescents.

While drowning is a leading cause of death worldwide, particularly in low- and middle-income countries, prevention is possible. Evidence shows that a range of interventions are effective at preventing drowning. Among others, these include the strategic use of barriers to control access to water, provision of safe places such as day care centres for pre-school children, and teaching school-age children basic swimming skills. Progress in other areas called for in this report includes better and more integrated flood risk management; improved boating, shipping and ferry regulations; and development of national water safety policies.

Advances in many of these areas are feasible for low- and middle-income countries, although they will need political will and technical support to achieve them. Some interventions, such as day care centres, provide benefits beyond drowning prevention.

Drowning also has important intersections with a range of major agendas, including climate change; mass migration, including of asylum seekers; and child and adolescent health. The multisectoral nature of drowning prevention demands improved coordination across various agendas and sectors.

While there is much to learn about drowning and drowning prevention, we must take proven, preventive action while research continues. This means urgently targeting vulnerable populations in exposed communities with strategies most likely to save lives.

Drowning has a similar burden today as diseases such as diarrhoea and measles in the 1970s and 1980s. These were daunting challenges that nonetheless were made the subject of concerted prevention efforts by national governments, nongovernmental organizations and international bodies. This approach can be successful today to reduce the global drowning burden.

Margaret Chan
Director-General,
World Health Organization

CONTRIBUTORS

EDITORIAL GUIDANCE

Editorial committee

David Meddings
Adnan A Hyder
Joan Ozanne-Smith
Aminur Rahman

Executive editor

David Meddings

Advisory committee

Stephen Beerman
Joost Bierens
Lauren S Blum
Anuradha Bose
Christine M Branche
Ruth Brenner
Alfredo Celis
Richard C Franklin
Jonathan P Guevarra
Olive Kobusingye
Michael Linnan
Kevin Moran
Linda Quan
AKM Fazlur Rahman
Frederick Rivara
Justin Scarr
Gordon S Smith

ACKNOWLEDGEMENTS

The World Health Organization would like to thank the members of the Editorial and Advisory committees whose contributions and peer review made the *Global report on drowning* possible.

The report also benefited from the contributions and review of a number of other people. In particular, acknowledgement is made to Angela Burton, who edited the report. Additional input and thoughtful reviews were contributed by Grant Baldwin, Jonathon Passmore and Carolyn Staines. Rebecca Bavinger, Jennifer Ellis, Kelly Henning and Kelly Larson from Bloomberg Philanthropies also contributed thoughtful reviews. Comments and contributions were also received from Erin Cassell, Milhar Fuazudeen, John Harding, Ashok Mahapatra, José Riera, Sumbul Rizvi, Katja Rytkoenen and Cecilia Scharp.

Other WHO staff who contributed to the report include Jonathan Abrahams, Rudi Coninx, Richard Johnston, Hyo-Jeong Kim, Etienne Krug, Rachel Mackenzie, Doris Ma Fat, Colin Mathers, Margie Peden and Florence Rusciano.

Finally the World Health Organization wishes to thank Bloomberg Philanthropies for its generous financial support for the development and publication of this report.

ABBREVIATIONS

CPR	Cardiopulmonary resuscitation
ICD	International Classification of Diseases
IMO	International Maritime Organization
ILS	International Life Saving Federation
NGO	Nongovernmental organization
UNHCR	United Nations High Commissioner for Refugees
UNICEF	United Nations Children's Fund
UNISDR	United Nations Office for Disaster Risk Reduction
WHO	World Health Organization

REGIONS OF THE WORLD HEALTH ORGANIZATION

AFRO	African Region
AMRO	Region of the Americas
EMRO	Eastern Mediterranean Region
EURO	European Region
SEARO	South-East Asia Region
WPRO	Western Pacific Region

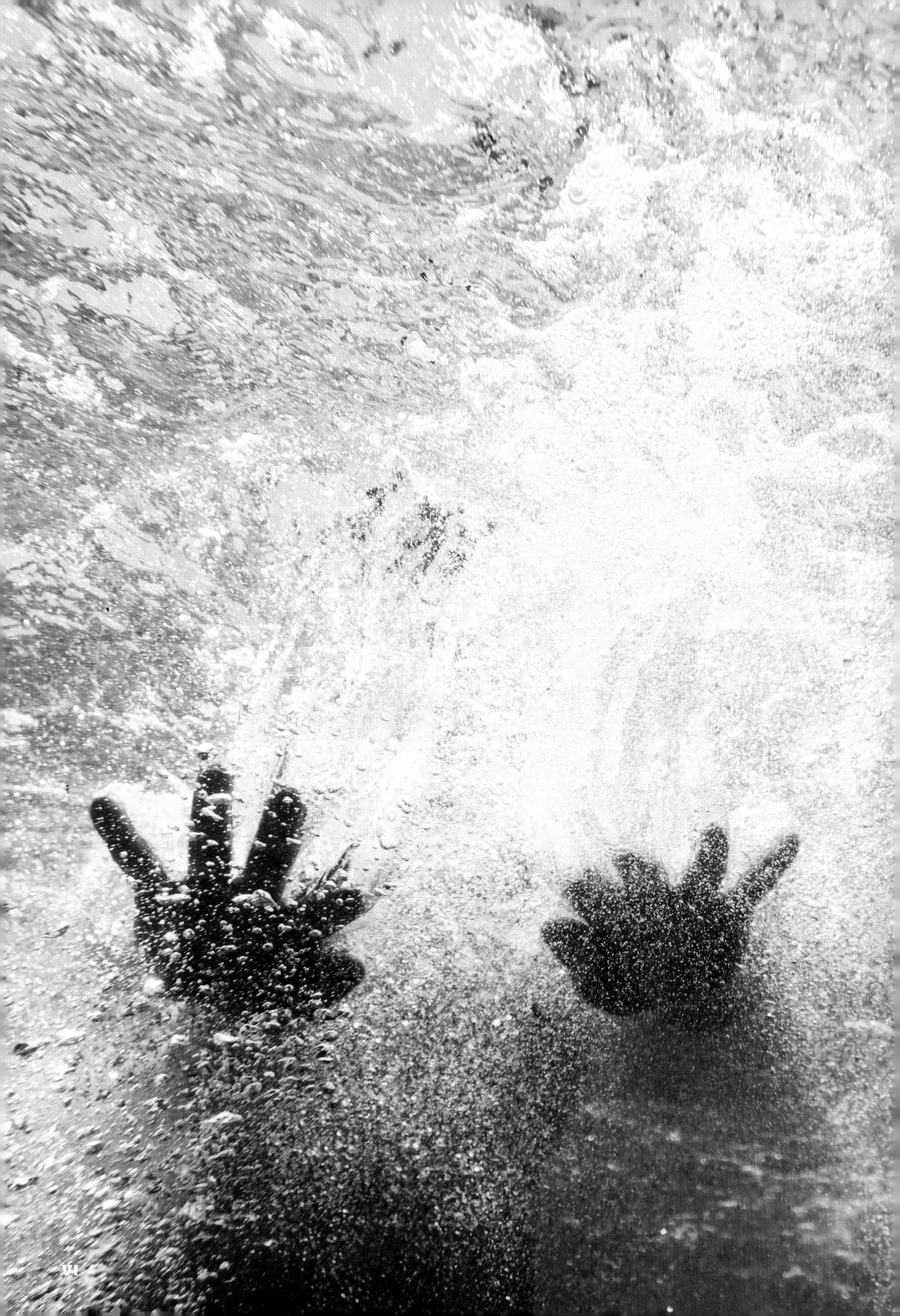

EXECUTIVE SUMMARY

Drowning is a serious and neglected public health threat claiming the lives of 372 000 people a year worldwide.

More than 90% of these deaths occur in low- and middle-income countries.

This death toll is almost two thirds that of malnutrition and well over half that of malaria – but unlike these public health challenges, there are no broad prevention efforts that target drowning.

EXECUTIVE SUMMARY

While this report addresses drowning across all countries and ages, the particularly high incidence of drowning in low- and middle-income countries and among children and young people makes these countries and groups a central focus.

OUR MESSAGE: PREVENTION IS VITAL

Once someone starts to drown, the outcome is often fatal. Unlike other injuries, survival is determined almost exclusively at the scene of the incident, and depends on two highly variable factors: how quickly the person is removed from the water, and how swiftly proper resuscitation is performed. **Prevention, therefore, is vital.**

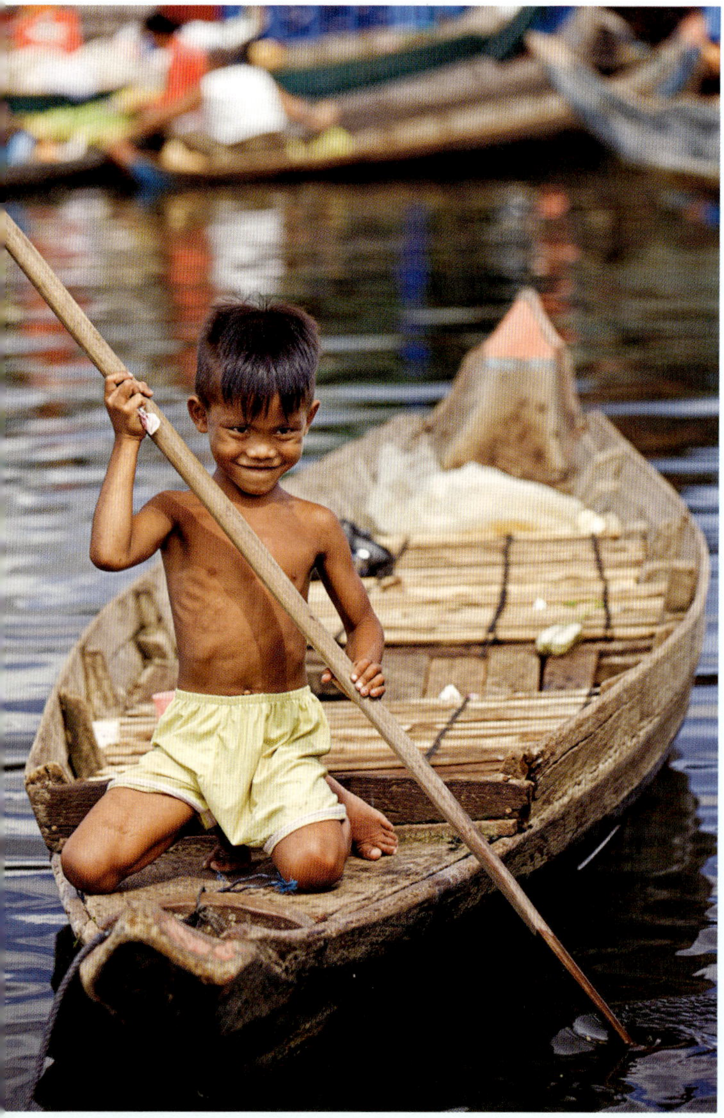

SECTION 1 DROWNING – A NEGLECTED PUBLIC HEALTH ISSUE

GLOBAL BURDEN

Alarmingly, drowning is among the 10 leading causes of death of children and young people in every region of the world, with children aged under 5 years disproportionately at risk and males twice as likely to drown as females. Over half of casualties are aged under 25 years. Income levels also have an impact – the overwhelming majority of drownings happen in low- and middle-income countries where people have close daily contact with water for work, transport and agriculture.

LIMITATIONS OF DATA

Data collection in many low- and middle-income countries is limited, hampering the planning, implementation and monitoring of drowning prevention measures. In addition, the way deaths are classified means the full extent of the world's drowning problem is underrepresented – statistics currently exclude intentional drowning (for example, suicide and homicide), as well as drowning deaths resulting from flood disasters and water transport incidents.[1] Data on non-fatal drownings, which could reveal something about the burden of serious injury and lifelong disability, are not routinely collected.

KEY RISK FACTORS

Lack of barriers controlling exposure to water bodies and lack of adequate, close supervision for infants and young children are a drowning risk, as are poor swim skills and low awareness of water dangers. In addition, high-risk behaviour, including consuming alcohol while engaging with water, is a risk among young people and adults. Other risk factors are transport on water and water crossings, lack of safe water supply, and flood disasters.

1 Using the International Classification of Diseases (ICD) 10, WHO's global drowning mortality estimates are based *only* on deaths where drowning is classified as the external cause of death (i.e. where drowning was the event that caused the death – for example, a child drowning in a well), and not those where drowning was only the consequence of another classified external cause of death (e.g. transport incident, suicide, homicide, flood disaster, etc.).

SECTION 2
TEN ACTIONS TO PREVENT DROWNING

High-income countries have reduced their drowning burden and some of the strategies used have been successfully adapted in low- and middle-income settings. Based on available evidence, Section 2 sets out 10 actions that can help prevent drowning.

COMMUNITY-BASED ACTION

1. Install barriers controlling access to water.

2. Provide safe places (for example, a crèche[2]) away from water for pre-school children, with capable child care.

3. Teach school-age children basic swimming, water safety and safe rescue skills.

4. Train bystanders in safe rescue and resuscitation.

5. Strengthen public awareness of drowning and highlight the vulnerability of children.

EFFECTIVE POLICIES AND LEGISLATION

6. Set and enforce safe boating, shipping and ferry regulations.

7. Build resilience and manage flood risks and other hazards locally and nationally.

8. Coordinate drowning prevention efforts with those of other sectors and agendas.

9. Develop a national water safety plan.

FURTHER RESEARCH

10. Address priority research questions with well-designed studies.

2 A crèche – also referred to as day care or a day care centre – is a place where young children are cared for during the day, usually while their parents are working.

SECTION 3
CONCLUSION AND RECOMMENDATIONS

Drowning is an important public health issue with major impacts on children and youth. Drowning is preventable. Proven strategies implemented at household, community and national level range from teaching basic swim skills and installing barriers that control exposure to water hazards, to providing safe spaces for children such as crèches and learning about safe rescue. Tailored to individual settings and risk groups, countries should take steps to improve data on drowning mortality and morbidity, and establish a national water safety plan.

Drowning is a multisectoral issue. Drowning prevention strategies have much in common with other public health agendas including safe water supply, rural development, disaster risk management and child health. More must be done to maximize these synergies – for example, village-based day care for pre-school children not only provides the early child development benefits associated with day care, it also prevents drowning and provides employment. Likewise, drowning risks could become a more clearly stated consideration of disaster risk management efforts in settings where flood disasters occur.

Given the multisectoral nature of drowning, a global partnership for drowning prevention should be established in order to serve as a policy and implementation leadership community for the issue of drowning prevention.

In summary, donors and governments must prioritize drowning prevention, and its integration with other public health agendas.

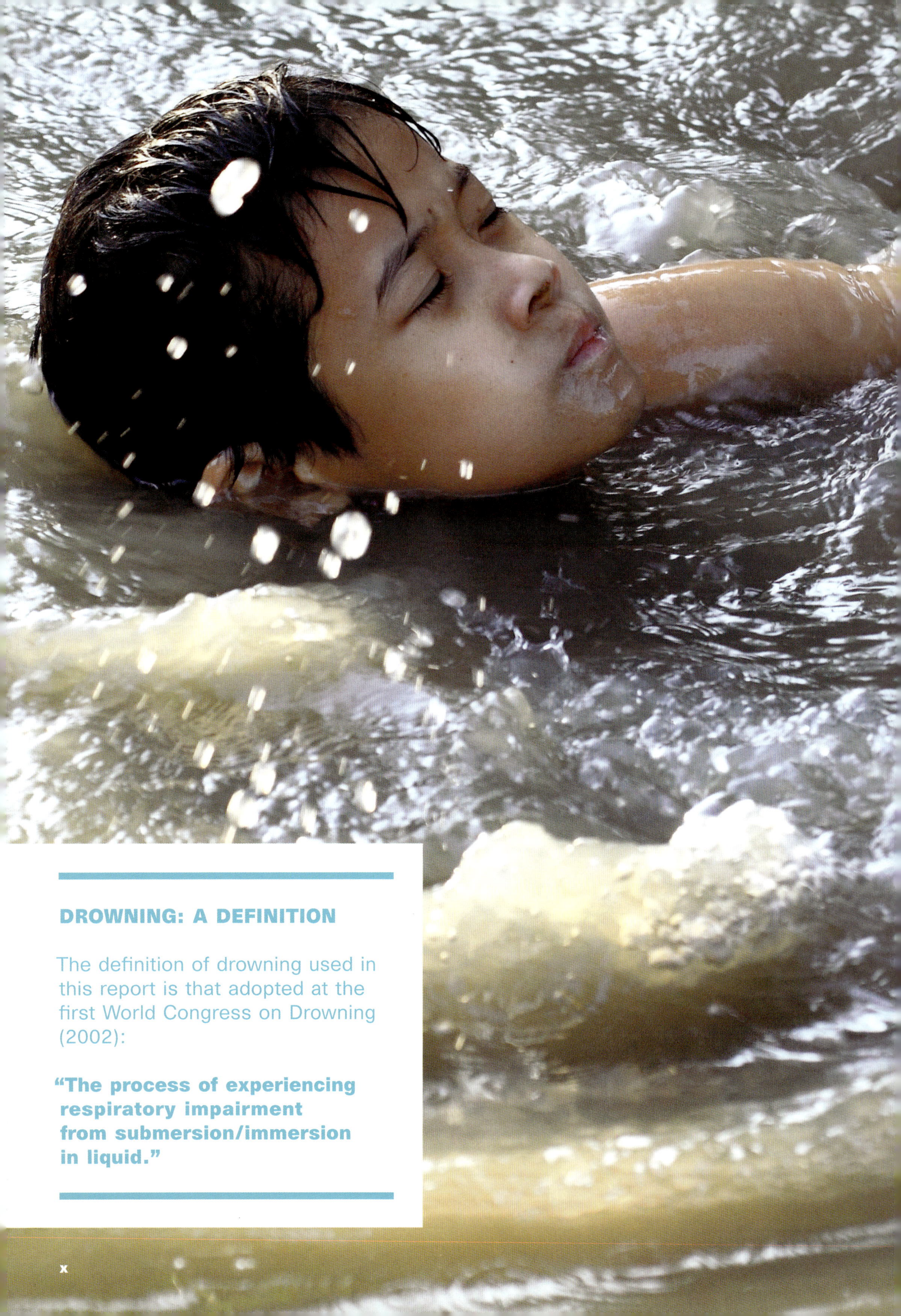

DROWNING: A DEFINITION

The definition of drowning used in this report is that adopted at the first World Congress on Drowning (2002):

"The process of experiencing respiratory impairment from submersion/immersion in liquid."

INTRODUCTION

There needs to be much more national and international attention focused on drowning, given the limited data available on its true scale and the heavy toll it takes on families, communities and economies.

This report aims to galvanize such attention and action by highlighting how preventable drowning is, and how collaboration across sectors – be it health and rural development, fisheries, maritime or disaster risk management – can save lives.

Section 1 sets out key estimates and risk factors for drowning based on the most recent data available to the World Health Organization (WHO).[3] It describes who is most affected, where, and how, and gives an overview of how tackling the drowning burden can be stepped up. Section 2 outlines 10 drowning prevention actions. Section 3 presents conclusions and recommendations.

3 See Appendix 2 for national death data reported to WHO, and WHO mortality estimates. Note these data are for deaths and do not include serious injury due to drowning (e.g. brain injury resulting from lack of oxygen).

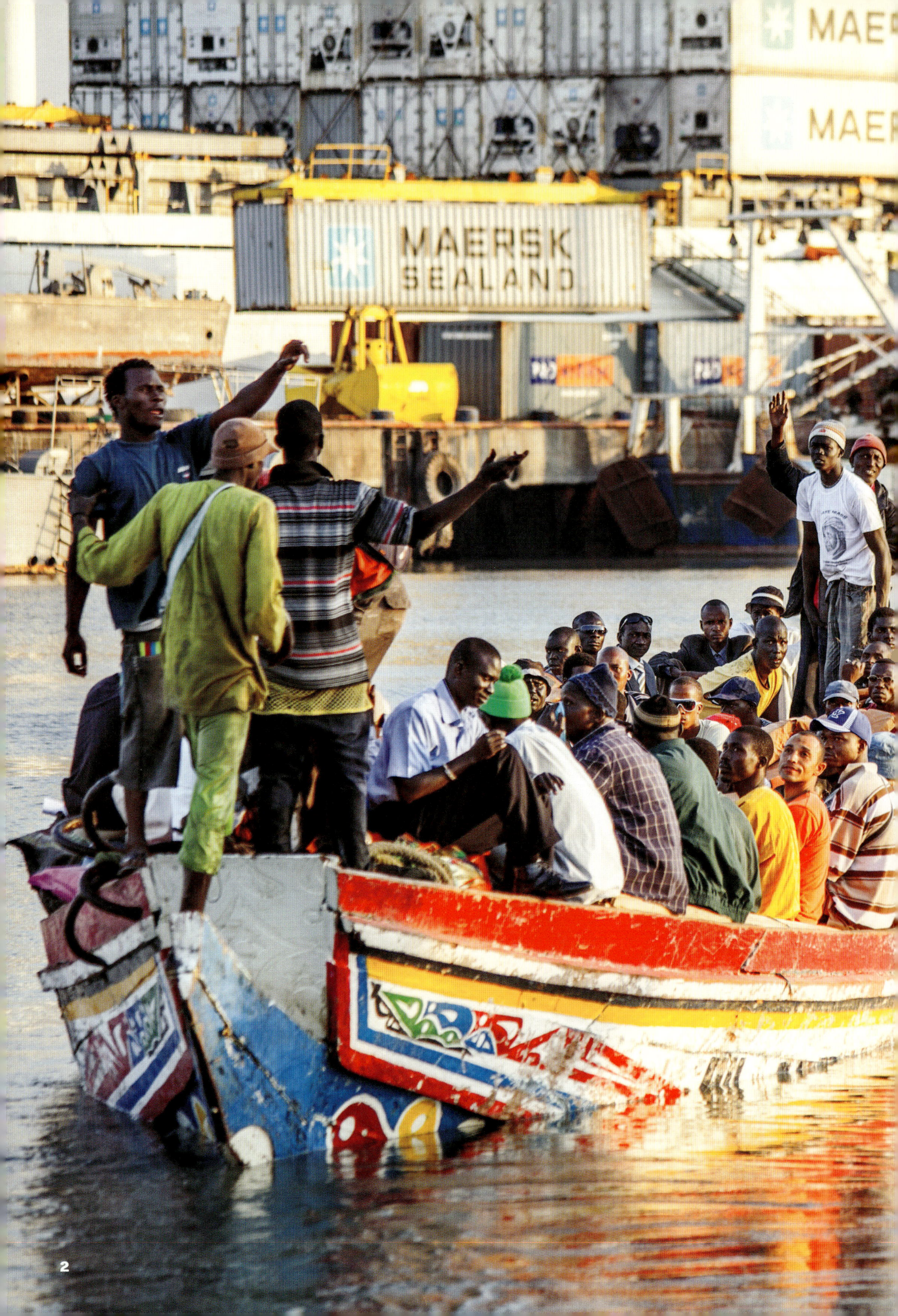
MAERSK
SEALAND

SECTION 1

DROWNING – A NEGLECTED PUBLIC HEALTH ISSUE

Relative to its global impact, drowning (fatal and non-fatal) is a vastly neglected area of public health. In 2012, an estimated 372 000 people died from drowning, making it the world's third leading unintentional injury killer.

THE FULL SCALE OF THE DROWNING PROBLEM IS UNKNOWN

The estimated death toll is all the more alarming because official data categorization methods for drowning exclude intentional drowning deaths (suicide or homicide) and drowning deaths caused by flood disasters and water transport incidents (including those where vessels carrying migrants, refugees and stateless people capsize during so-called irregular transport on water).

Data from high-income countries suggest these categorization methods result in significant underrepresentation of the full drowning toll by up to 50% in some high-income countries.[4] Survey data from a number of low- and middle-income countries contrast markedly with WHO estimates – some suggest a level four or five times higher than the WHO estimated drowning rate.[5]

Other factors obscuring the full scale of global drowning include poor data collection systems, the fact that many drowning victims never reach a medical facility where their death may have been recorded, and the rapid burial of drowning victims (for cultural reasons) that leads to deaths remaining unreported.

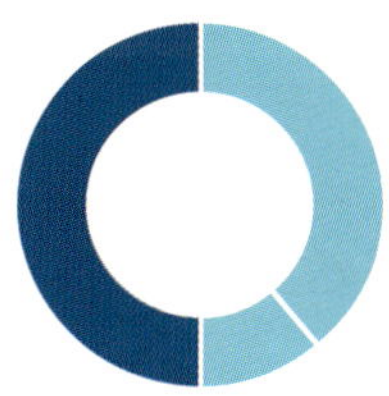

39–50%

The increase in drowning deaths in countries such as Australia, Finland and the USA if deaths recorded under other causes (e.g. water transport incident) were classed as drowning deaths.

Source: Linnan M et al. Child Drowning: Evidence for a newly recognized cause of child mortality in low- and middle-income countries and its prevention. Working Paper 2012-07, Special Series on Child Injury No. 2. Florence, UNICEF Office of Research, 2012.

4 Lunetta P et al. Unintentional drowning in Finland 1970–2000: A population-based study. International Journal of Epidemiology. 2004;33(5):1053–1063.
5 Peden M et al, eds. World report on child injury prevention 2008. Geneva: World Health Organization and UNICEF; 2008.

BOX 1

DROWNING ACCOUNTS FOR 43% OF DEATHS AMONG CHILDREN AGED 1–4 YEARS, BANGLADESH

The Bangladesh Demographic Health Survey 2011 says the country's *"absolute risk of death (per 1000 live births) declined substantially between 2004 and 2011 for most causes, except for deaths due to drowning... Diarrhoea, which has always been considered a major cause of child morbidity and mortality in Bangladesh, is now responsible for only 2% of under-five deaths. Although deaths from infectious disease have declined, drowning has emerged as a key cause of death, especially among children aged 12 to 59 months (43%)."*

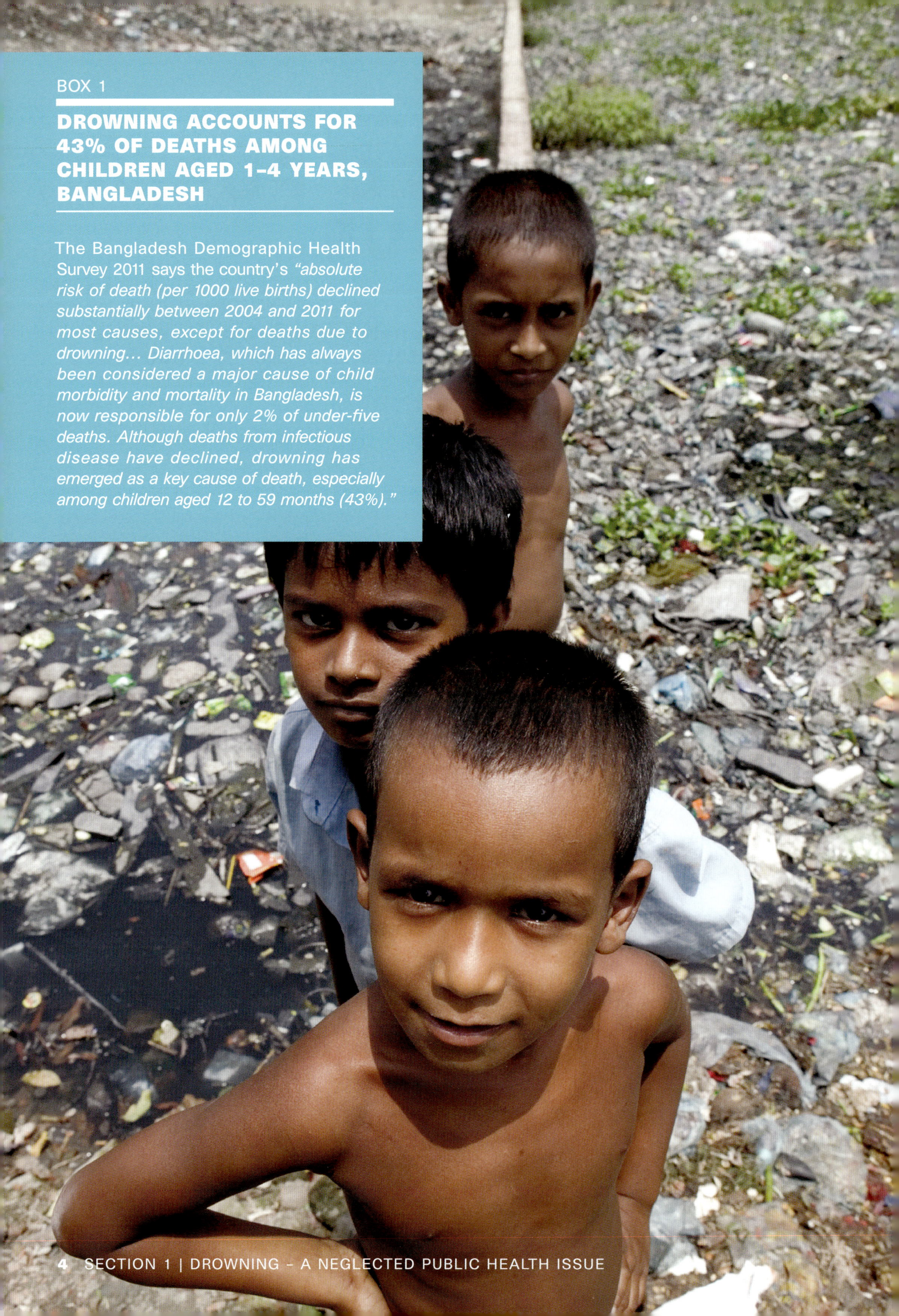

NEGLECT EXTENDS TO PREVENTION EFFORTS, POLICY AND RESEARCH

Poor-quality drowning data have contributed to a neglect of drowning prevention research. While there has been some success globally in focusing attention on drowning prevention, prevention efforts have mainly targeted recreational settings in high-income countries - not the day-to-day settings in low- and middle-income countries where the vast majority of drowning occurs, and where action is most urgently needed.

Many successful drowning prevention strategies from high-income country settings are unlikely to be appropriate for low- and middle-income settings, so it is vital that tackling drowning prevention in low- and middle-income countries is done using strategies tailored to the local context.

DROWNING NEEDS TARGETED ATTENTION LIKE OTHER PUBLIC HEALTH ISSUES

The success that targeted attention can bring to tackling public health issues is clear - in many low- and middle-income countries, childhood killer diseases have declined dramatically over the past three decades. However, drowning has seen no such decline - in Bangladesh, drowning now accounts for 43% of deaths among children aged 1-4 (see Box 1). And in the Matlab area, a subdistrict of Bangladesh with a well-established demographic health surveillance system, this figure exceeds 60% (see Figure 1).

FIGURE 1

EMERGENCE OF DROWNING AS THE LEADING KILLER OF CHILDREN AGED 1–4 YEARS, MATLAB, BANGLADESH

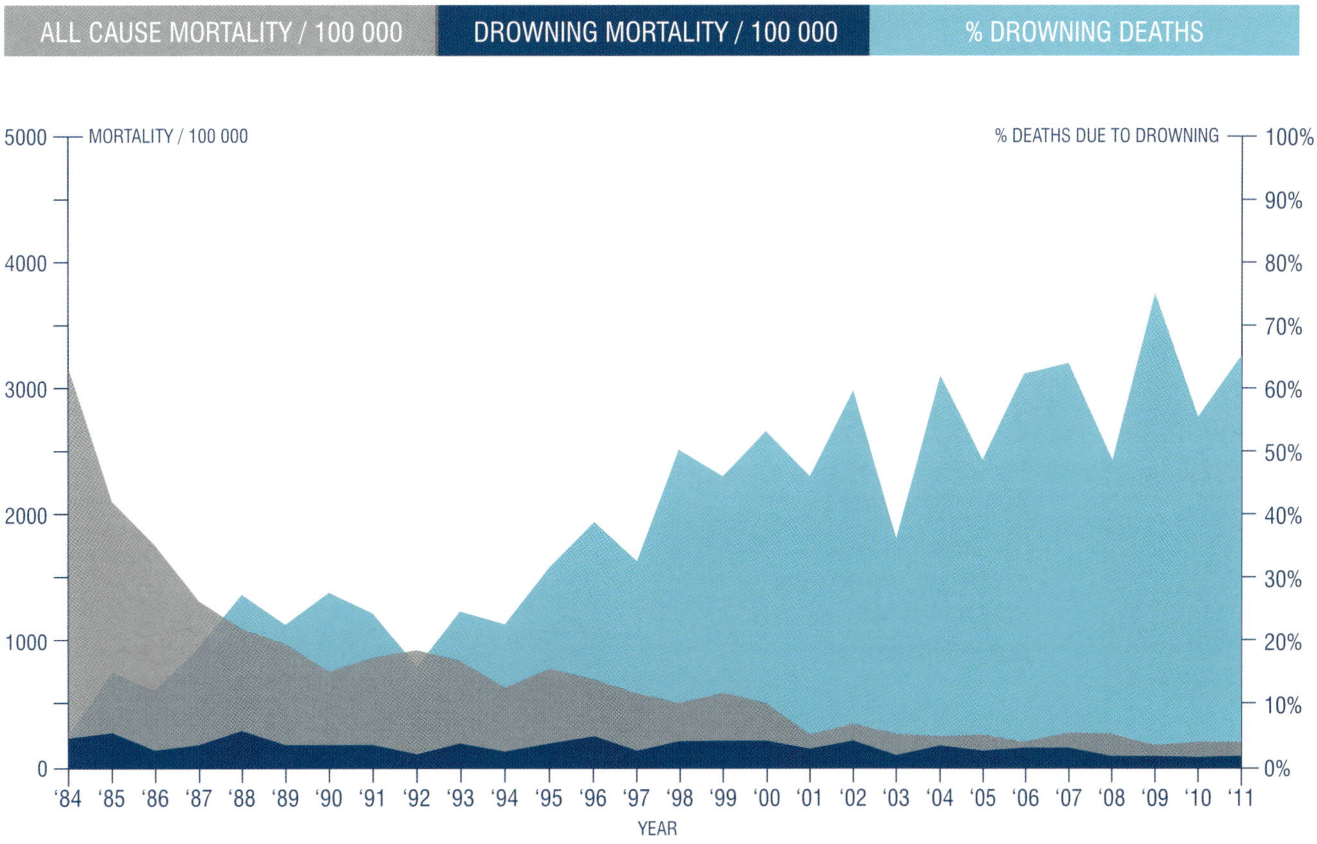

DROWNING KEY FACTS

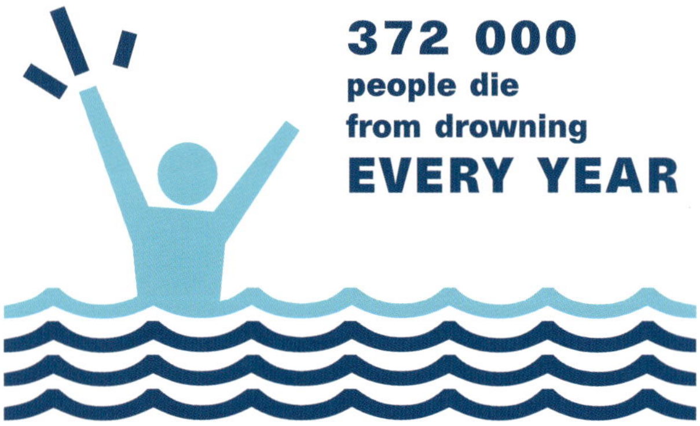

372 000 people die from drowning **EVERY YEAR**

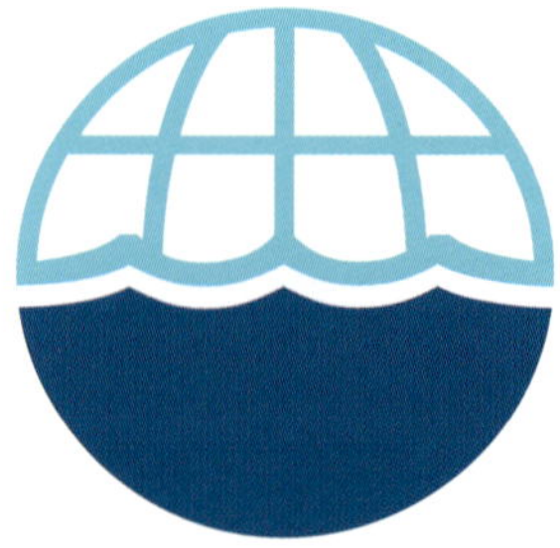

Globally, **OVER HALF** of all drowning deaths are among those aged **UNDER 25 YEARS**

There are approximately **42 DROWNING DEATHS EVERY HOUR,** every day

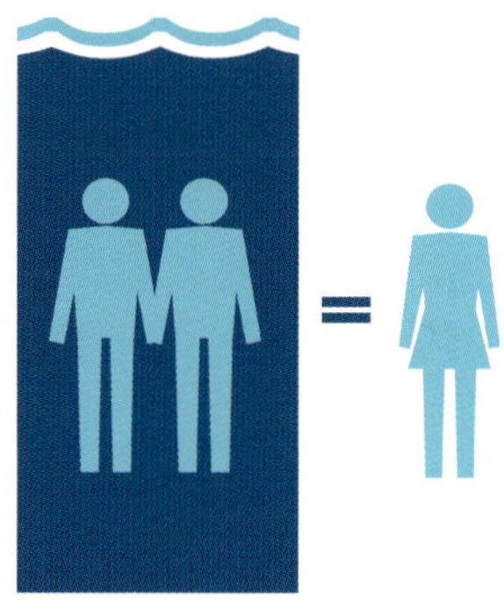

MALES ARE TWICE AS LIKELY to drown as females

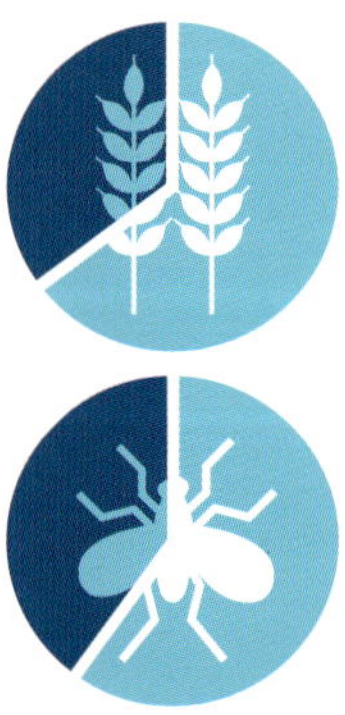

The drowning death toll is almost **TWO THIRDS** that of malnutrition and well **OVER HALF** that of malaria

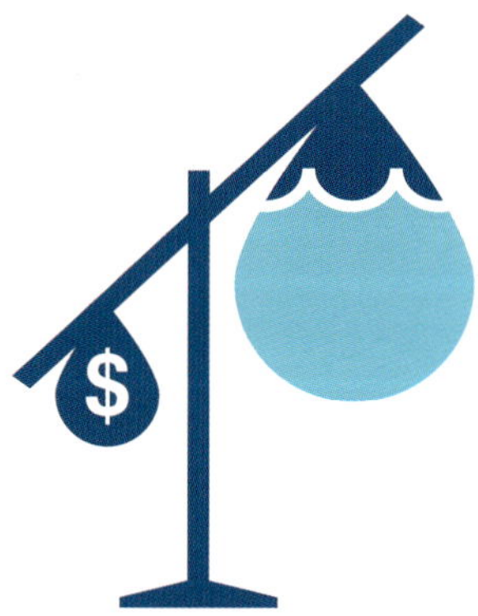

Drowning rates in low- and middle-income countries are **OVER THREE TIMES HIGHER** than in high-income countries

Drowning is one of the **10 LEADING CAUSES OF DEATH** for people aged 1–24 years in every region of the world (see Figure 2)

Alcohol use around water is an **IMPORTANT RISK FACTOR** for drowning in many countries, especially for adolescents and adults[6]

6 Ahlm K, Saveman B, Björnstig U. Drowning deaths in Sweden with emphasis on the presence of alcohol and drugs – a retrospective study, 1992-2009. BMC Public Health. 2013;Mar 11;13:216.

FIGURE 2

RANK OF DROWNING AMONG 10 LEADING CAUSES OF DEATH BY REGION AND AGE GROUP

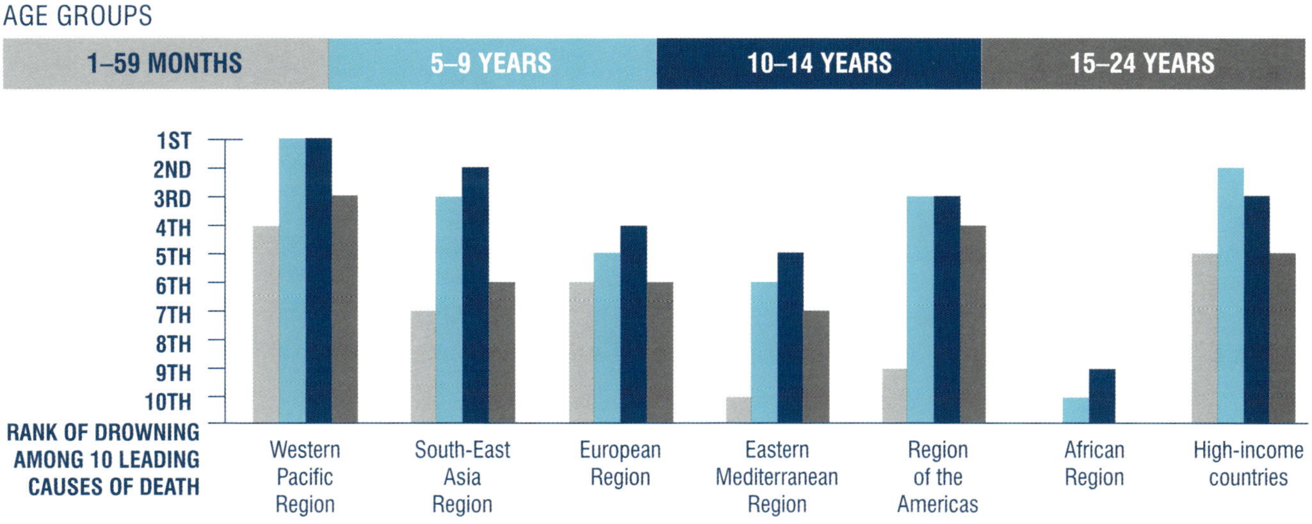

Note: Data for all high-income countries appears as 'High-income countries'. All WHO regions provided show ranking for only the low- and middle-income countries within those regions.

FIGURE 3

DROWNING AS A LEADING CAUSE OF DEATH AMONG 1–14 YEAR OLDS, SELECTED COUNTRIES

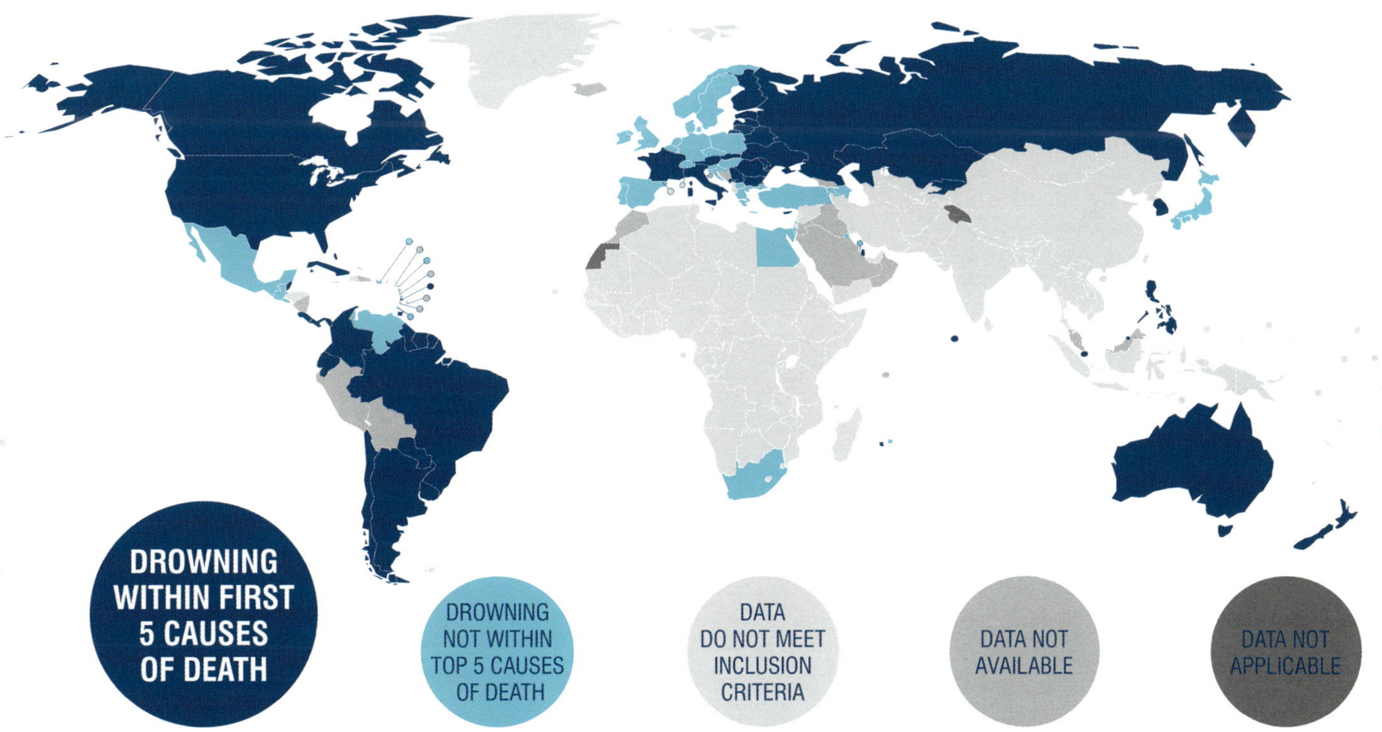

Analysis of mortality data submitted to WHO shows **drowning is one of the top five causes of death for people aged 1–14 years for 48 of the 85 countries** where data meet inclusion criteria (see Figure 3).[7]

7 Mortality data for countries were considered if they met the following criteria: estimated coverage of national deaths of 70% or more; ill-defined causes of death less than 20%; 10 or more deaths in the 1–14 year old age group; and data available from 2007 or later.

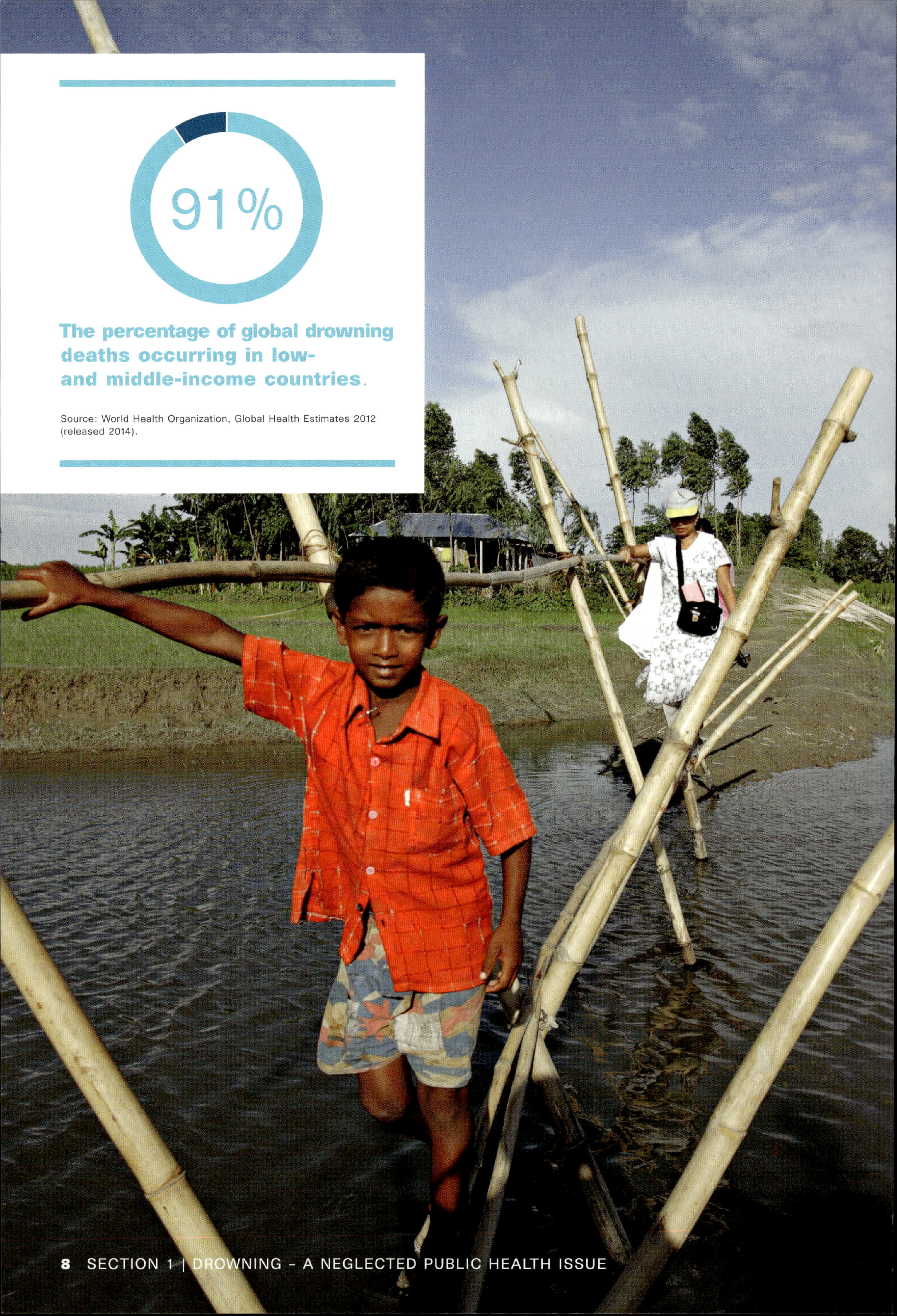

The percentage of global drowning deaths occurring in low- and middle-income countries.

Source: World Health Organization, Global Health Estimates 2012 (released 2014).

WHAT ARE THE RISKS?

Drowning happens in many different ways, and needs a range of prevention strategies to target the biggest risks. The main risk factors are:

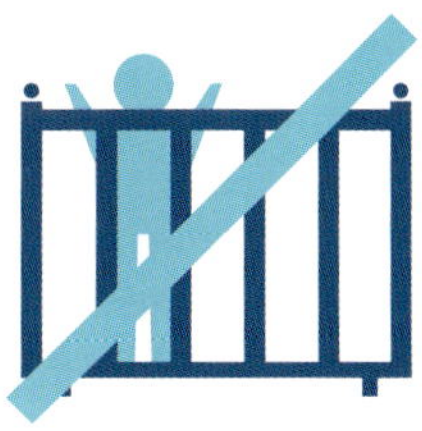

Lack of physical barriers between people and water, particularly close to home

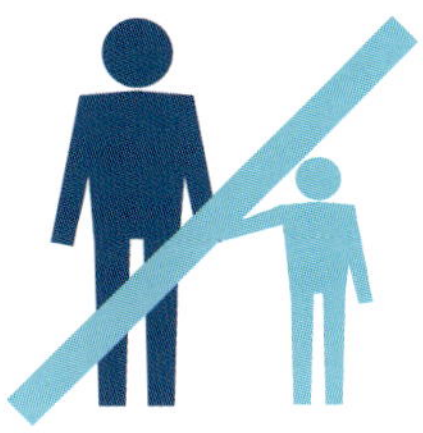

Lack of (or inadequate) supervision of young children

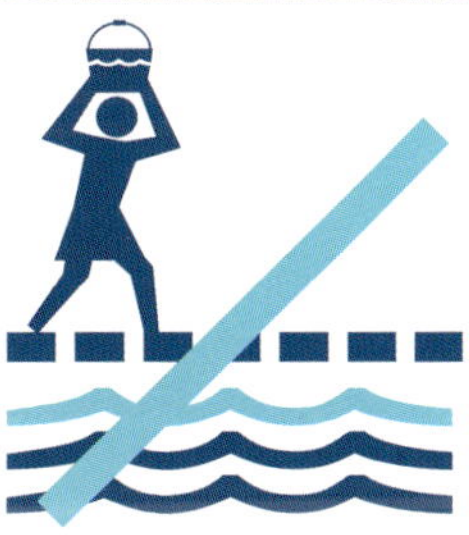

Uncovered or unprotected water supplies and lack of safe water crossings

Lack of water safety awareness and risky behaviour around water, such as swimming alone

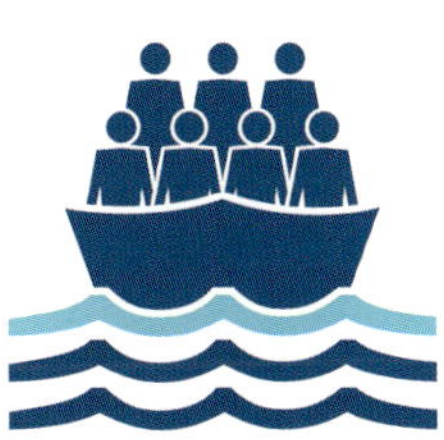

Travelling on water, especially on overcrowded or poorly maintained vessels

Flood disasters, whether from extreme rainfall, storm surges, tsunamis or cyclones

WHO IS AT RISK?

PEAK DROWNING RATES ARE AMONG CHILDREN

Globally, the highest drowning rates are among children aged 1–4 years, followed by children aged 5–9 years. Worldwide, males are twice as likely to drown as females.

In the Western Pacific Region, children aged 5–14 years die more frequently from drowning than from any other cause, meaning drowning deaths outnumber those caused by road traffic crashes, congenital anomalies, leukaemia, lower respiratory infections, epilepsy, dengue and meningitis (see Figure 2).[8]

CHILDREN'S VULNERABILITY CHANGES WITH AGE

- Children aged under 12 months are relatively immobile and entirely dependent on caregivers. They can drown very quickly and in very little water, and in water containers that may not be perceived as risks (for example, in a bucket or a toilet).
- Children who are mobile but too young to recognize danger or to get out of water are at risk, especially in the absence of barriers and capable supervision.
- Adolescents tend to be less supervised and are more likely to engage in risky behaviour around water, including consuming alcohol.

8 The Convention on the Rights of the Child defines childhood as ending on the 18th birthday, but because health data collection systems typically report data for 5-year age groups, the statistics in this report refer to children as those aged under 19 years. In this report, age ranges are always indicated in tables and figures.

DROWNING HITS THE POOR AND MARGINALISED

Regional drowning rates in low- and middle-income countries are up to 3.4 times greater than those in high-income countries (see Figure 4).

Regardless of a country's economic development, drowning often hits the poorest and least-educated people who live in rural settings (especially around water), and communities with the least resources to safely adapt to the risks around them. Drowning rates are also disproportionately high among minority populations in places where overall drowning rates are low, including in high-income countries.[9]

9 According to the *World report on child injury prevention* (2008), in high-income countries there are large differences in fatal drowning rates between population subgroups, with an increased risk of between two and four times for children and young people from racial ethnic minority groups. Suggested explanations include difference in swimming ability and experience in the water, lack of opportunities to learn to swim and lack of supervision in environments where such population groups are at high-risk.

DROWNING DESTROYS LIVES AND LIVELIHOODS

Fatal drowning is an abrupt and tragic loss of a loved one - a child, a mother, a father. And when many people drown at once, as in flood disasters, or when a ferry capsizes, entire villages and communities are shattered.

The economic cost of lives lost is also high, and while difficult to quantify globally, national-level estimates for Australia, Canada and the United States of America (USA) range from US$ 85 million to US$ 4.1 billion per year.

In high-income countries in particular, those who survive drowning but are left with catastrophic brain damage and disability create a potentially overwhelming challenge of care and financial cost for families. At the same time, lack of adequate medical care in low- and middle-income countries means those surviving but disabled by drowning often do not live long.

FIGURE 4

AGE-STANDARDIZED DROWNING DEATHS PER 100 000 POPULATION, BY REGION AND INCOME LEVEL

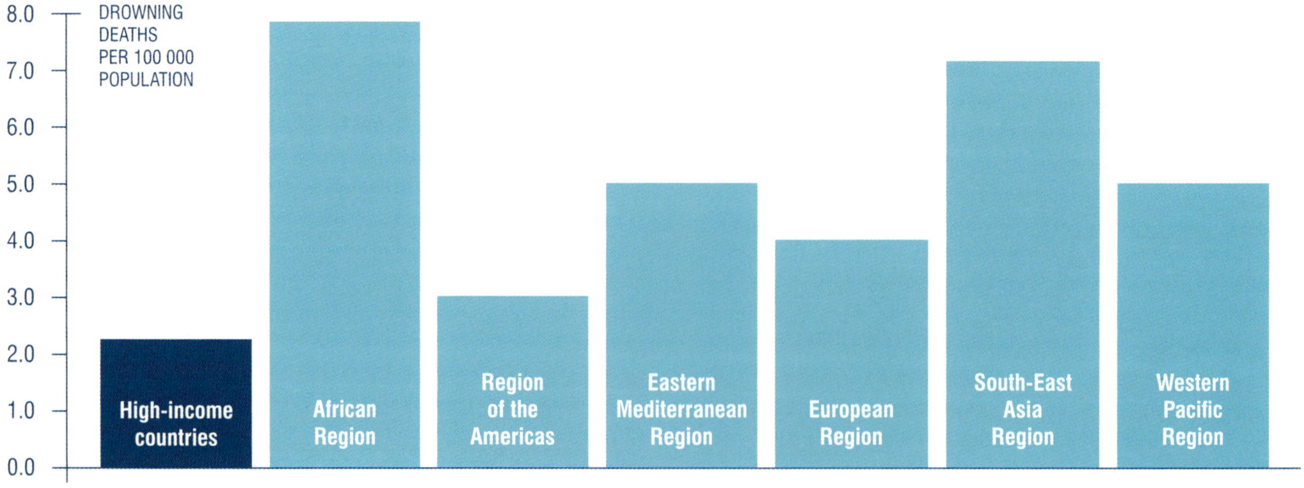

Note: Data for all high-income countries appears as 'High-income countries'. All WHO regions provided show ranking for only the low- and middle-income countries within those regions.

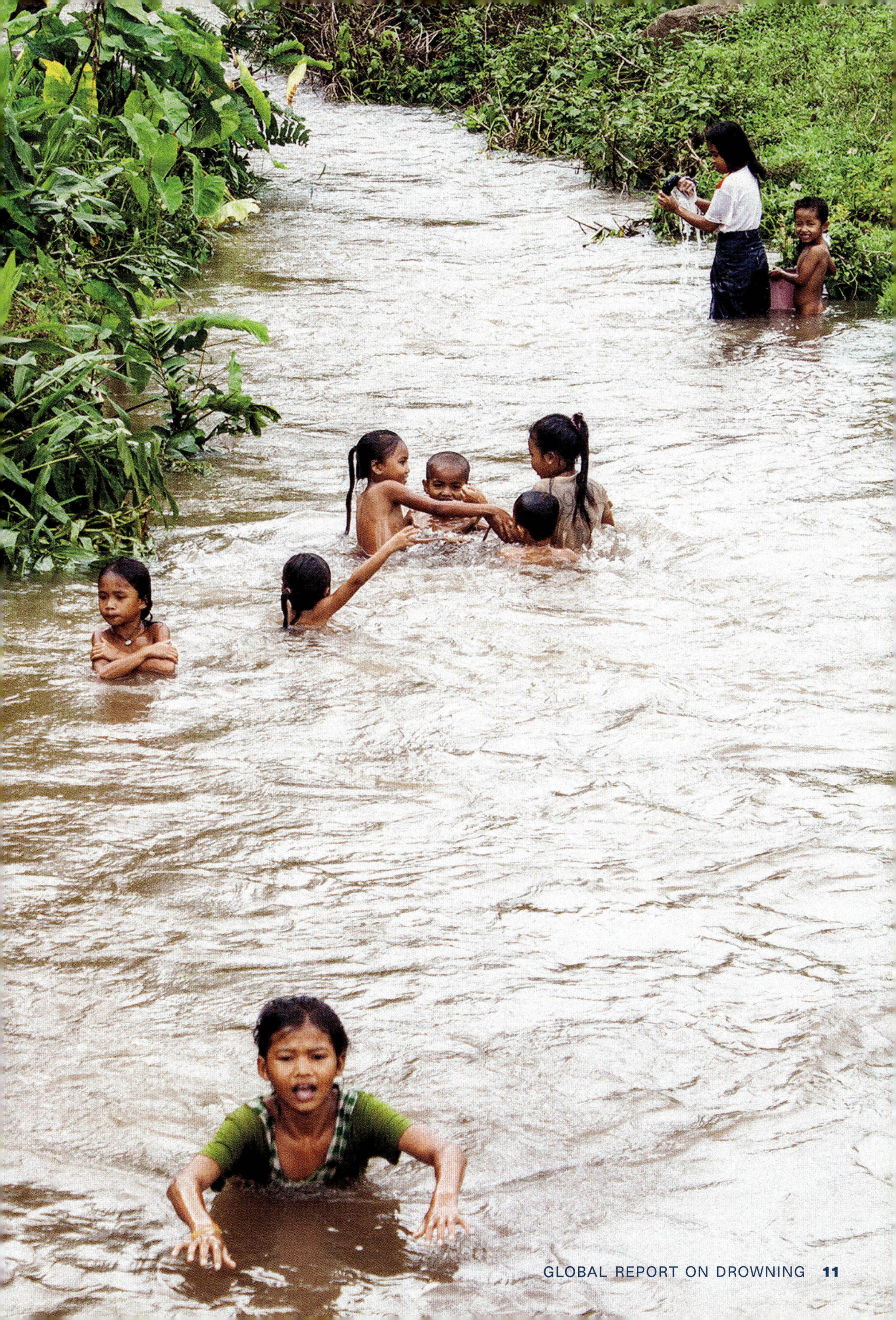

WHERE ARE THE RISKS?

Bucket, bathtub, pond or pool: wherever there is water, there is the threat of drowning

Even in countries with large coastlines such as Australia, Canada, New Zealand and Viet Nam, most drowning happens inland. Whether in a bucket, bathtub, pond or pool, almost all water is a risk for drowning - especially where young children are concerned.

In Bangladesh, a national survey found 80% of drowning among children aged under 5 years happened within 20 metres of the family home - mainly in ponds, followed by ditches and water containers (see Figure 5). Older children and adults drown further away from home, typically in natural water bodies, often while working, travelling or collecting water.

A similar study in the rural community of Kaniyambadi, in Vellore, India, found that nearly 90% of drowning deaths among children aged 1-12 years involved water in a pot, well or pond.[10]

LIVING AROUND WATER

People in low- and middle-income countries interact with water very differently to those in high-income countries, and the general level of economic and social development in low- and middle-income countries means exposure to water is riskier.

- **Collecting water**
  Just under half the world's population have no access to piped water, meaning water holes, wells or surface water are the only water sources for drinking, washing, cooking and daily household chores.[11]

- **Living near water**
  Lack of barriers or signs around water hazards such as unsafe crossings, open wells, uncovered manholes and ditches in low- and middle-income countries poses a risk. In low- and middle-income countries, many homes in these settings are on lakes or river banks - some are built over the water - and this, along with poor flood disaster protection, puts local people at greater risk.

- **Travelling on water**
  Daily commuting and journeys made by migrants or asylum seekers often take place on overcrowded and unsafe vessels that lack safety equipment or are operated by personnel not trained to deal with transport incidents or high-seas navigation. Personnel under the influence of alcohol or drugs are also a risk.

- **Working on or around water**
  Small-scale fishing is estimated to employ around 37 million people worldwide - around 90% are in Asia.[12] Reducing drowning risk for these and others who earn their living on or around water requires adequate enforcement of safety standards and equipment, and warning services such as weather alerts.

- **Flood disasters**
  The number of people exposed to hazards is rising with the increased frequency and severity of flood disasters, and unplanned urbanization. Drowning risks increase with floods, particularly in low- and middle-income countries where people live in flood-prone areas and the ability to warn, evacuate, or protect communities from floods is weak or only just developing. Between 1980 and 2009 there were over 500 000 estimated deaths from floods and 2.8 billion people affected by floods worldwide (excluding tsunamis).

10 Bose A, George K, Joseph A. Drowning in childhood: a population-based study. Indian Pediatrics. 2000;37:80-83.
11 Joint Monitoring Programme (JMP) for Water Supply [online database]. Geneva: WHO/UNICEF (http://www.wssinfo.org/data-estimates/tables/, accessed 19 May, 2014).
12 Small-scale fisheries around the world. FAO Fisheries and Aquaculture Department [website]. Rome: Food and Agriculture Organization (http://www.fao.org/fishery/ssf/world/en, cited 3 April 2014).

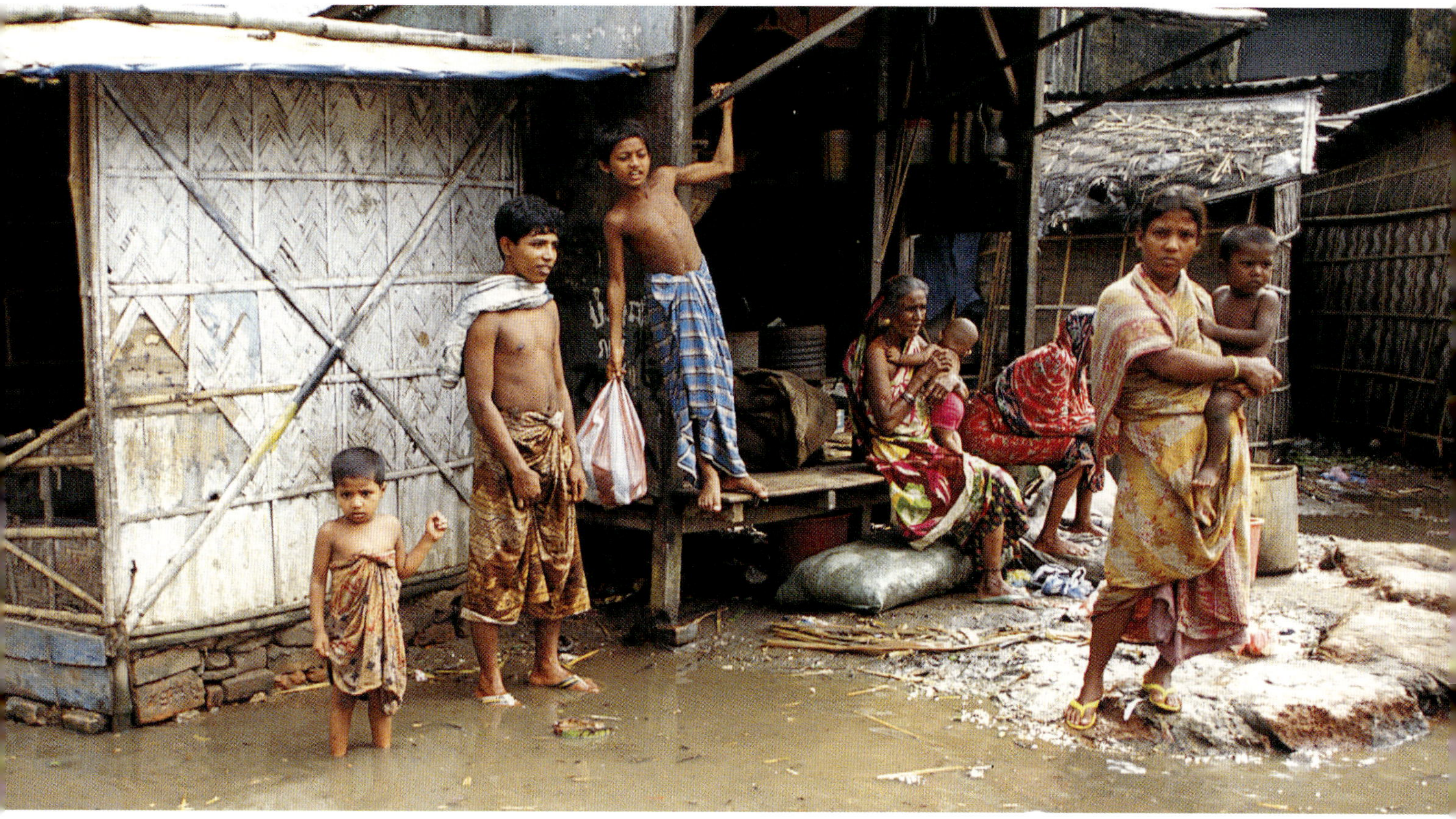

FIGURE 5

PLACE OF DROWNING OF BANGLADESHI CHILDREN AGED UNDER 5 YEARS

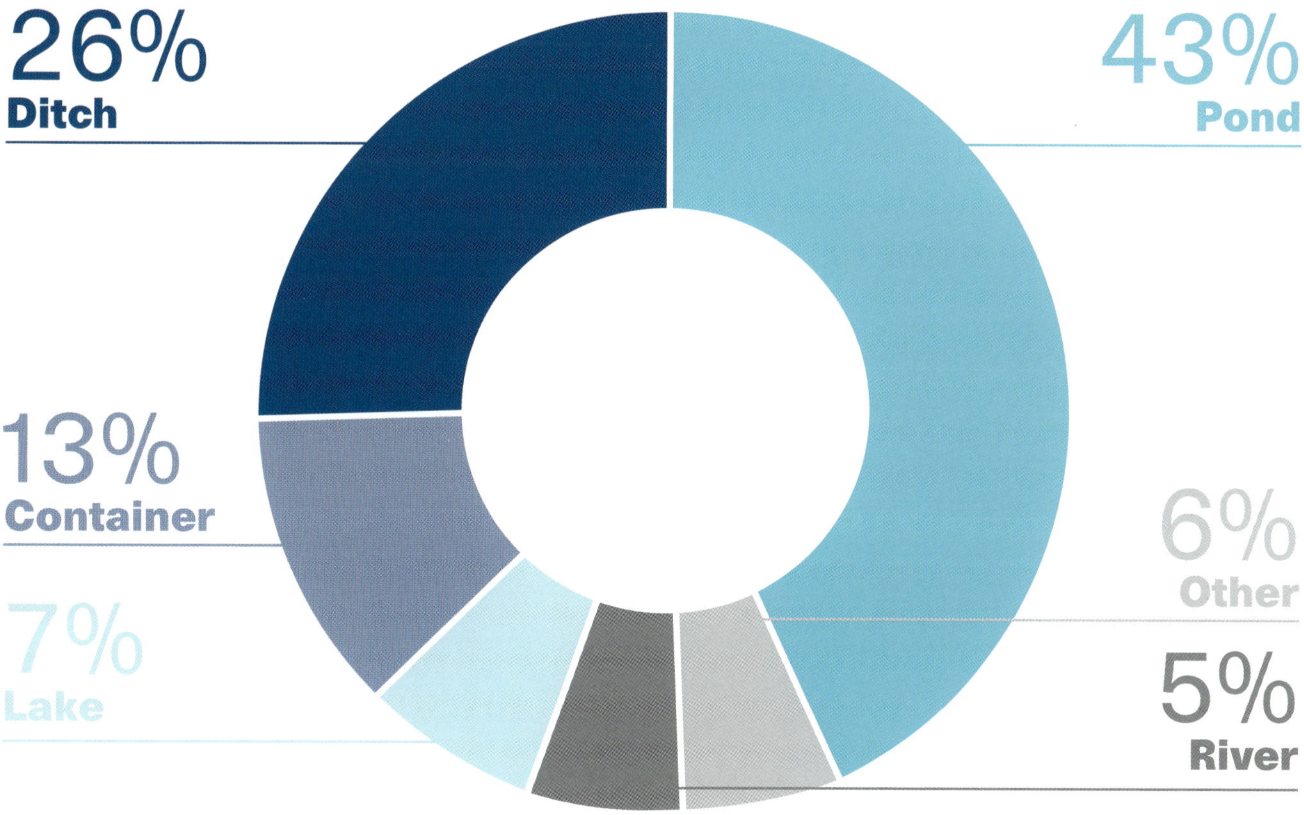

Source: Rahman A et al. Analysis of the childhood fatal drowning situation in Bangladesh: exploring prevention measures for low-income countries. Injury Prevention. 2009;15:75-79.

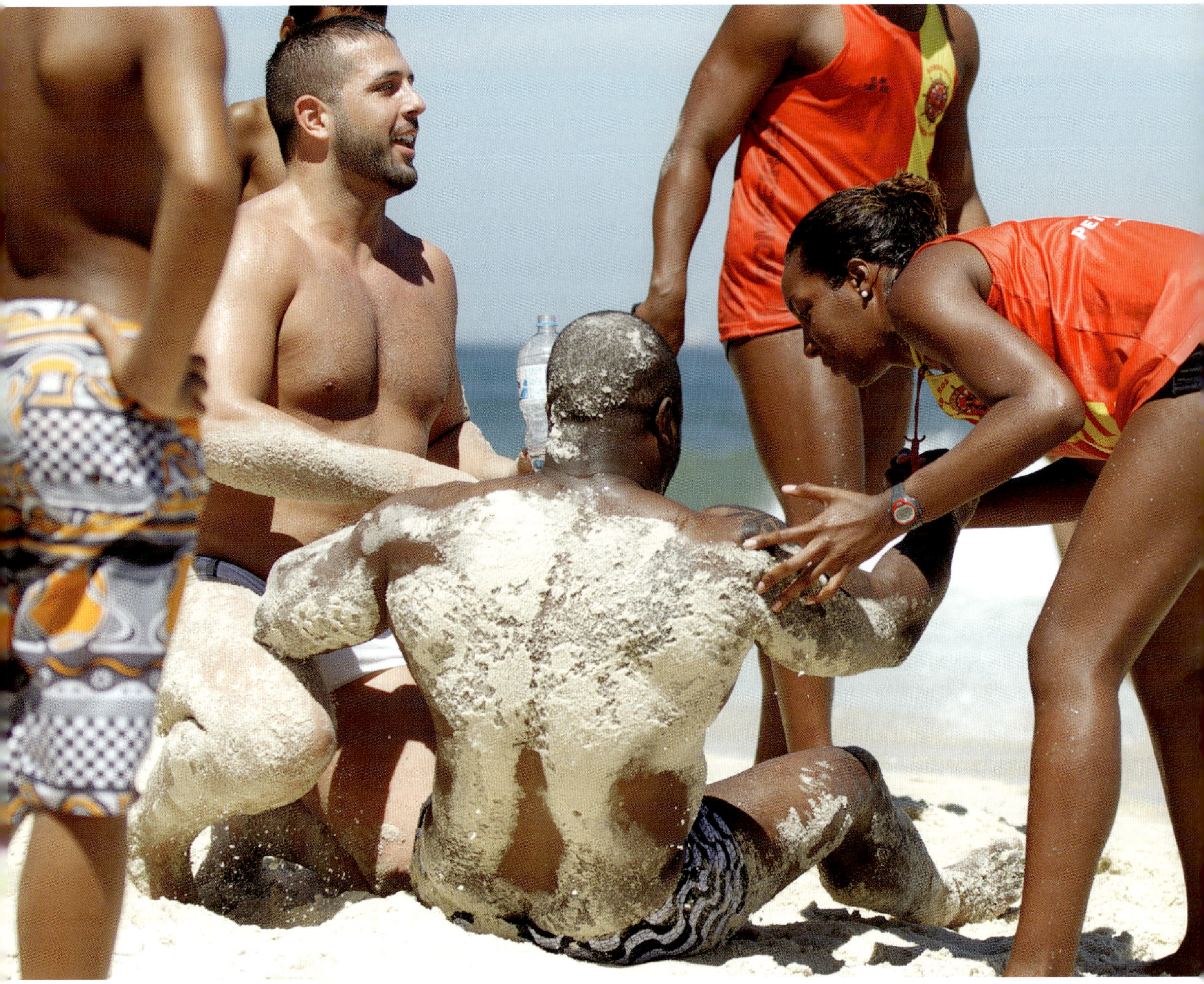

WHERE ASSISTANCE IS LIMITED

Rescue and resuscitation must be done immediately at the scene of the incident if it is to be effective, making it highly desirable that the skills to perform rescue and resuscitation of drowning victims are present in as much of the population as possible.

But establishing programmes to instil these skills in low- and middle-income countries requires a certain set of conditions, including generally high education levels, a culture of good Samaritanism and legal protection for those attempting rescue and resuscitation. Lack of these conditions poses a significant obstacle to the establishment and effective function of such programmes in low- and middle-income countries.

Added to this, traditional responses such as forcibly pushing the stomach or rubbing the victim with salt or ashes can cause harm, as they delay or prevent effective cardiopulmonary resuscitation (CPR) as may other cultural or religious beliefs. Transport to a medical facility for further treatment may also be severely limited because of distance or cost.

HOW CAN WE REDUCE THE THREAT OF DROWNING?

Drowning can be prevented through targeted prevention strategies, improved community infrastructure (water supply, bridges, levees etc.), public awareness, appropriate policies and legislation, and research that refines what is seen as best practice and that identifies new drowning prevention measures.

Strategies such as these have worked in high-income countries and some low- and middle-income countries - scaling up these approaches will bring further gains.

ADAPT SUCCESSFUL STRATEGIES FOR DIFFERENT SETTINGS

Drowning rates show long-term declines in high-income countries. Some of these reductions are likely the result of the provision of piped water, reduced exposure to open water, and better literacy and economic development, but other factors such as safety standards, policies and legislation have also played a role. Measures readily achievable in low-income settings include:

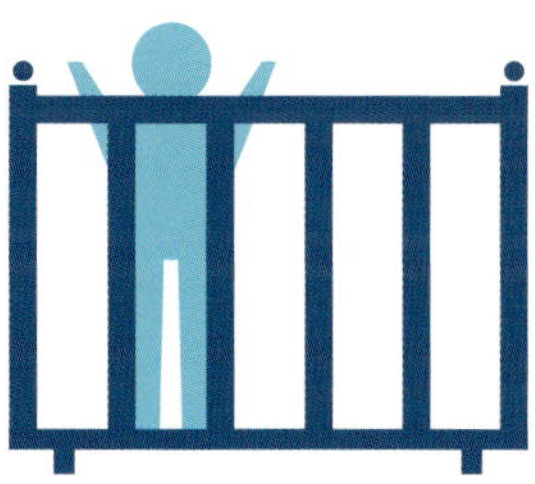

Reduced exposure to water hazards through strategic use of barriers

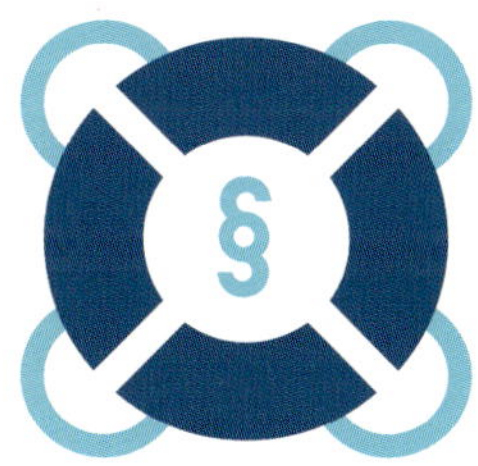

Comprehensive boating regulations and enforcement

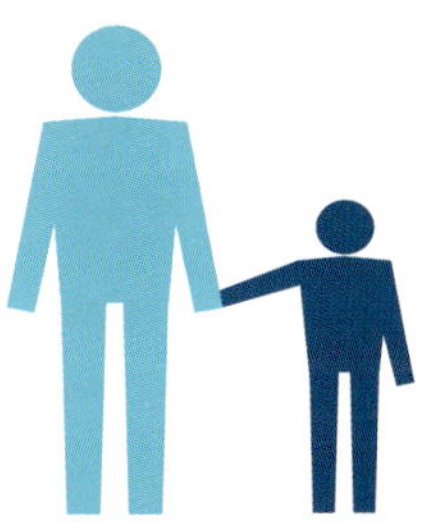

Close and capable adult supervision for young children

Signage and designation of hazardous water bodies

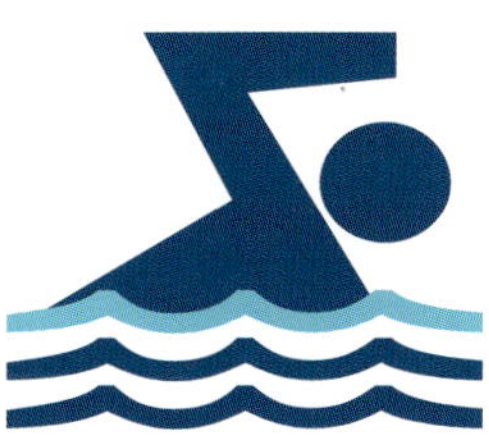

Improved swimming and water safety skills

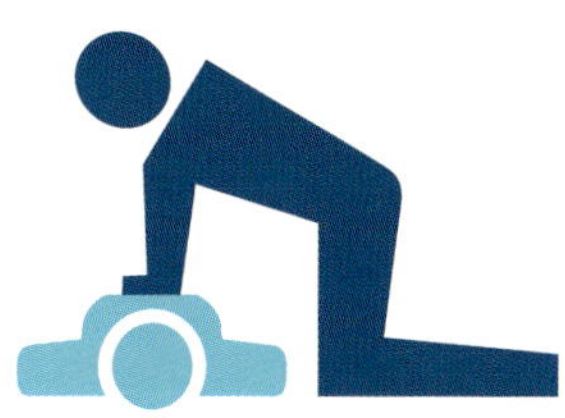

Timely rescue and resuscitation by a trained bystander or lifesaver through mouth-to-mouth resuscitation and chest compression when needed

Requirements for use of personal flotation devices (PFDs, see Box 2)

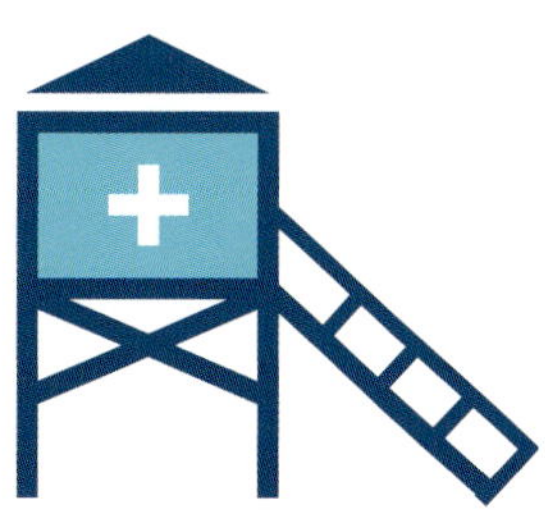

Supervision of recreational swimming areas

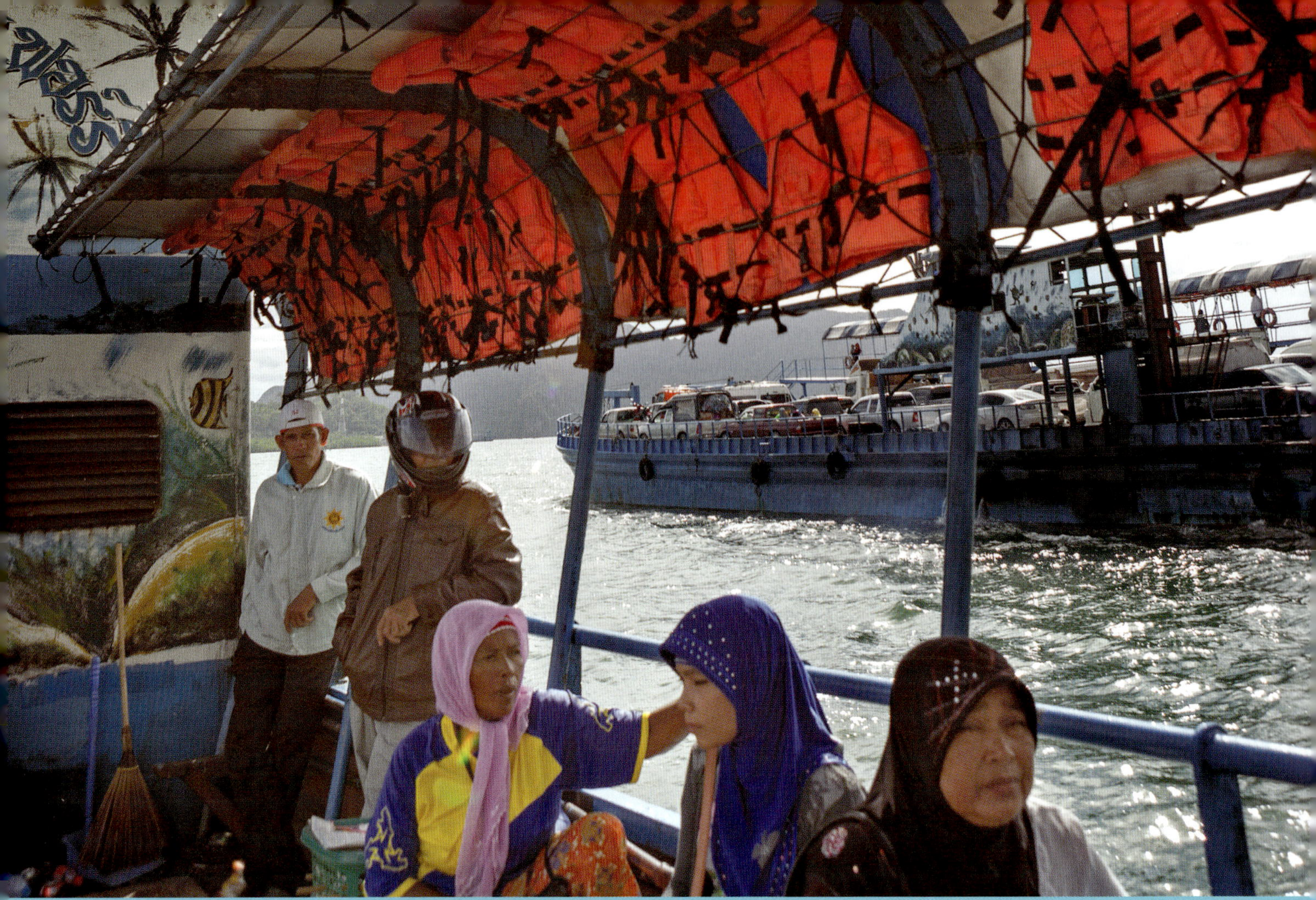

BOX 2

PERSONAL FLOTATION DEVICES (PFDS)

The term 'personal flotation device' (PFD) covers flotation devices such as lifejackets, as well as buoyancy devices designed to keep the wearer afloat (but that do not meet the higher performance requirements for lifejackets, which are designed to prevent drowning at sea). PFDs are considered appropriate for use by children, recreational boaters and water-sports participants undertaking activities in calm waters, close to the shore or close to help from rescuers.

Some governments require all recreational vessels to carry one wearable PFD (of a specified type) for each person on board but authorities and water safety bodies generally advocate that PFDs be worn by boaters to protect against unexpected entry into the water. The findings of a recent study of United States Coast Guard records comparing risk of drowning death for PFD wearers and non-wearers indicated that 50% of recreational boating drowning deaths may be prevented by wearing an appropriate PFD. Two Australian states have introduced regulations mandating PFD wearing for recreational boaters. A before-after observational study of the effectiveness of these in one state found the regulations were associated with a significant increase (from 22% to 63%) in PFD wearing. A subsequent study found the regulations were effective in reducing drowning deaths among all recreational boaters, to 59 recreational boating drowning deaths occurring in the six-year pre-legislation period compared to 16 in the 5-year post-legislation period.

Sources:

Cummings P, Mueller BA, Quan L. Association between wearing a personal floatation device and death by drowning among recreational boaters: a matched cohort analysis of United States Coast Guard data, Injury Prevention. 2011;17:156-9.

Cassell E, Newstead S. Did compulsory wear regulations increase personal flotation device (PFD) use by boaters in small power recreational vessels? A before-after observational study conducted in Victoria, Australia. Injury Prevention. 2014; 2 June. doi:10.1136/injuryprev-2014-041170.

Bugeja L, Cassell E, Brodie LR, Walter SJ. Effectiveness of the 2005 compulsory personal flotation device (PFD) wearing regulations in reducing drowning deaths among recreational boaters in Victoria, Australia. Injury Prevention. 2014; 23 June. doi: 10.1136/injuryprev-2014-041169.

BUILD ON SUCCESSES IN LOW- AND MIDDLE-INCOME COUNTRIES

There is increasing evidence of effective drowning prevention programmes in low- and middle-income countries. The SwimSafe programme – a regional, basic swim skills training programme operating in Bangladesh, Thailand and Viet Nam – is one example of this. A study of SwimSafe Bangladesh demonstrated a significant reduction in drowning following basic swimming and water safety training for children aged 4–12 years and the establishment of child care centres for children aged 1–5 years (see page 22). Initial cost-effectiveness of these strategies, individually and combined, compare favourably with other interventions to reduce child mortality.

INTEGRATE DROWNING PREVENTION INTO THE LOCAL SETTING

Understanding the way communities live around water is critical to developing and implementing effective drowning prevention programmes and policies (see Box 3). This is particularly important in low- and middle-income settings, where many livelihoods depend on water, where there are fewer (and often less-safe) water crossings and bridges, and where there is a heavy dependence on boats and ferries – making everyday life riskier than in high-income settings.

MAKE DROWNING PREVENTION PART OF A MULTISECTORAL APPROACH

A wide range of sectors influence drowning risk, including fisheries, maritime transport, disaster risk management, health, and rural development. Because of this, it is important that drowning prevention programmes and activities are multisectoral. Coordination across sectors can be of particular benefit in low- and middle-income countries, where doing more to prevent drowning will likely require efforts across a range of sectors.

BOX 3

WORKING WITH THE COMMUNITY TO PREVENT DROWNING, THE PHILIPPINES

A drowning prevention pilot project in Lucao village, Dagupan City, Philippines, engaged villagers in researching and choosing suitable drowning prevention measures. The project – culturally appropriate and site-specific – identified local risks by reviewing drowning mortality records, holding key informant interviews, focus group discussions and community 'walk-throughs'.

Risk factors identified were proximity to bodies of water without barriers, inadequate child supervision, lack of information and awareness of prevention strategies and lack of drowning prevention programmes. The measures implemented through the community's newly developed drowning prevention committee included community education sessions, redesigning community wells, developing playpens, using barriers around water and training community workers to deliver safety messages and teach people CPR.

Source: Guevarra JP, Franklin RC, Basilio JA, Orbillo LL, Go JJ. Child drowning prevention in the Philippines: the beginning of a conversation. International Journal of Injury Control and Safety Promotion. doi: 10.1080/17457300.2014.912235

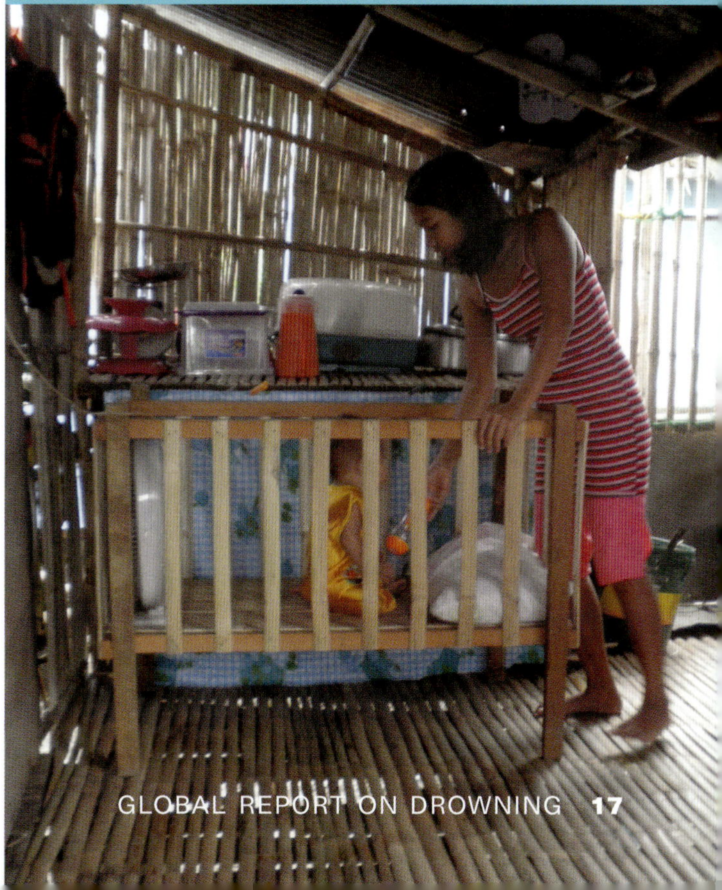

SECTION 2

TEN ACTIONS TO PREVENT DROWNING

The 10 actions outlined in this section are based on available evidence and are deemed to be effective, feasible and scalable. Complementary measures such as drawing on best-practice models, using social media and communication to raise public awareness, and adapting interventions to suit local contexts (for example, making barriers from locally sourced materials) are important in ensuring these strategies are effectively implemented.

In addition, in resource-poor settings where educational levels are low, it is important to understand how people perceive drowning before introducing interventions, including what local people see as the cause of drowning and appropriate ways to treat and prevent it. Findings should guide how actions are implemented.

Our 10 actions fall into three categories:

COMMUNITY-BASED ACTION

1

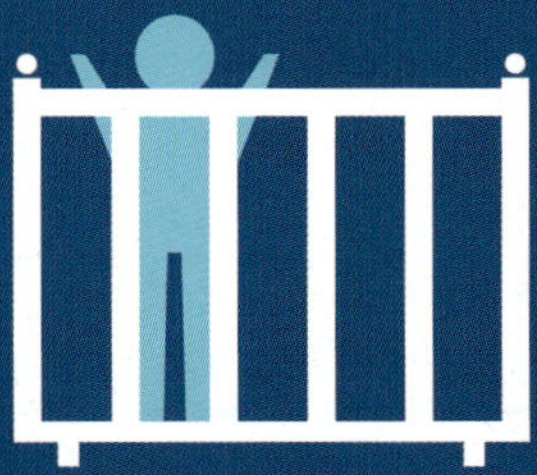

Install barriers controlling access to water

2

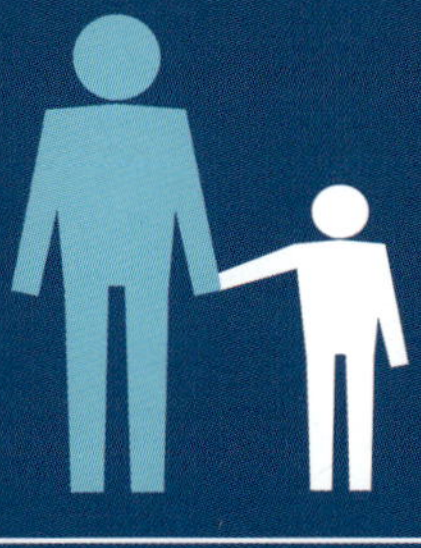

Provide safe places (for example, a crèche) away from water for pre-school children, with capable child care

3

Teach school-age children basic swimming, water safety and safe rescue skills

4

Train bystanders in safe rescue and resuscitation

5

Strengthen public awareness and highlight the vulnerability of children

EFFECTIVE POLICIES AND LEGISLATION

6

Set and enforce safe boating, shipping and ferry regulations

7

Build resilience and manage flood risks and other hazards locally and nationally

8

Coordinate drowning prevention efforts with those of other sectors and agendas

9

Develop a national water safety plan

FURTHER RESEARCH

10

Address priority research questions with well-designed studies

COMMUNITY-BASED ACTION

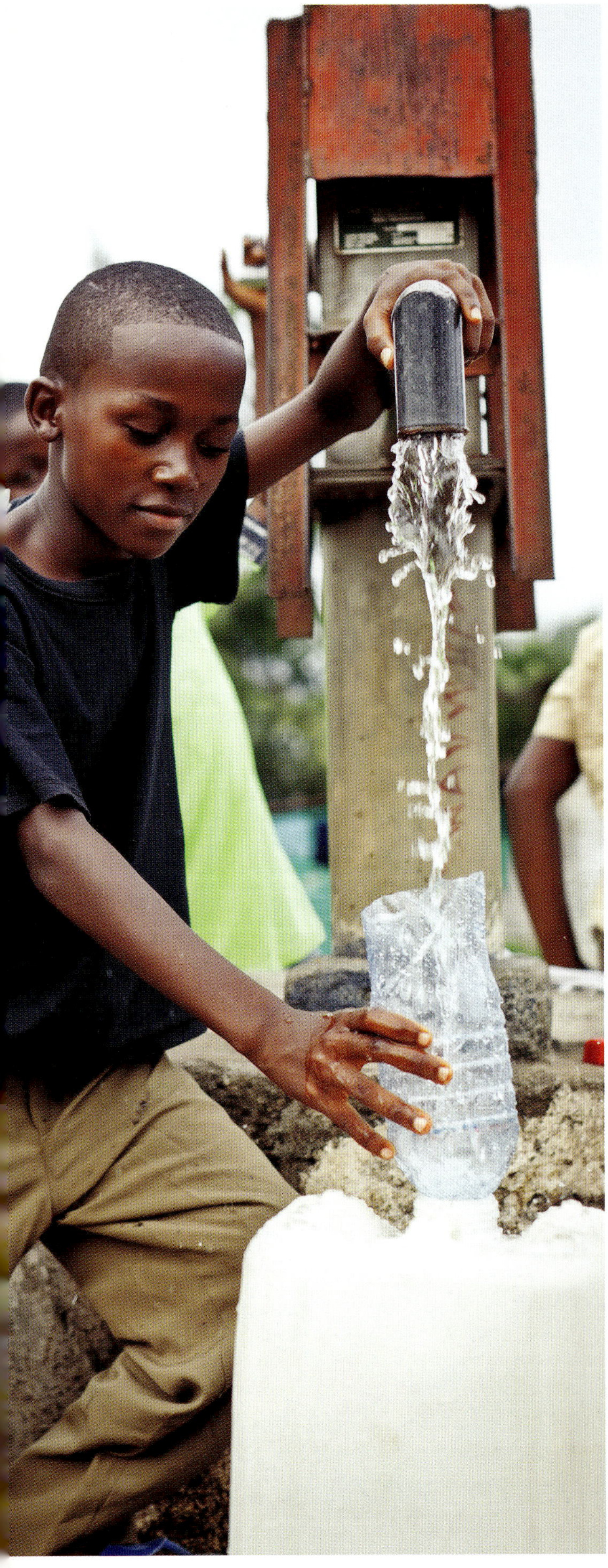

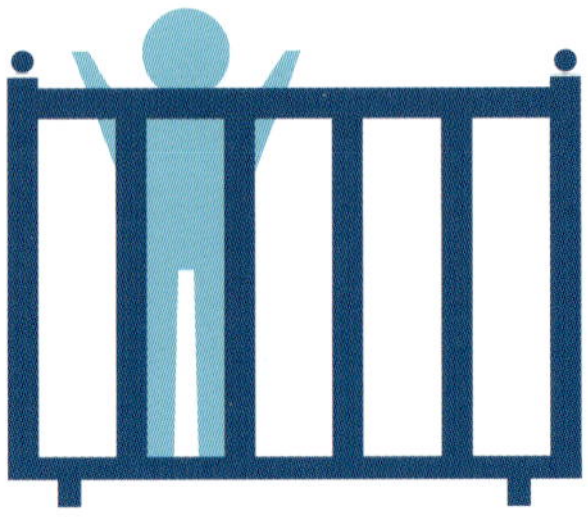

1 INSTALL BARRIERS CONTROLLING ACCESS TO WATER

Placing barriers strategically so access to water hazards is limited or more tightly controlled reduces exposure and drowning risk. While seemingly a straightforward task, care must be taken to ensure barriers are practical, sustainable, and create no further risk by their use.

Barrier approaches to prevent drowning include:

- **covering wells and cisterns** (water tanks). The use of a pump (manual, electrical or other) helps keep the water source covered while water is drawn.
- **using doorway barriers and playpens**.[13] The use of barriers should not replace the care or attention of a capable, supervising adult, or run the risk of the child being trapped.
- **fencing swimming pools** with four-sided, child-resistant fences and self-closing gates with safety latches.
- **legislating** for the implementation and enforcement of policies, standards and building codes to support these measures.

13 A playpen is a portable, four-sided enclosure in which a baby or young child can be safely placed without constant supervision.

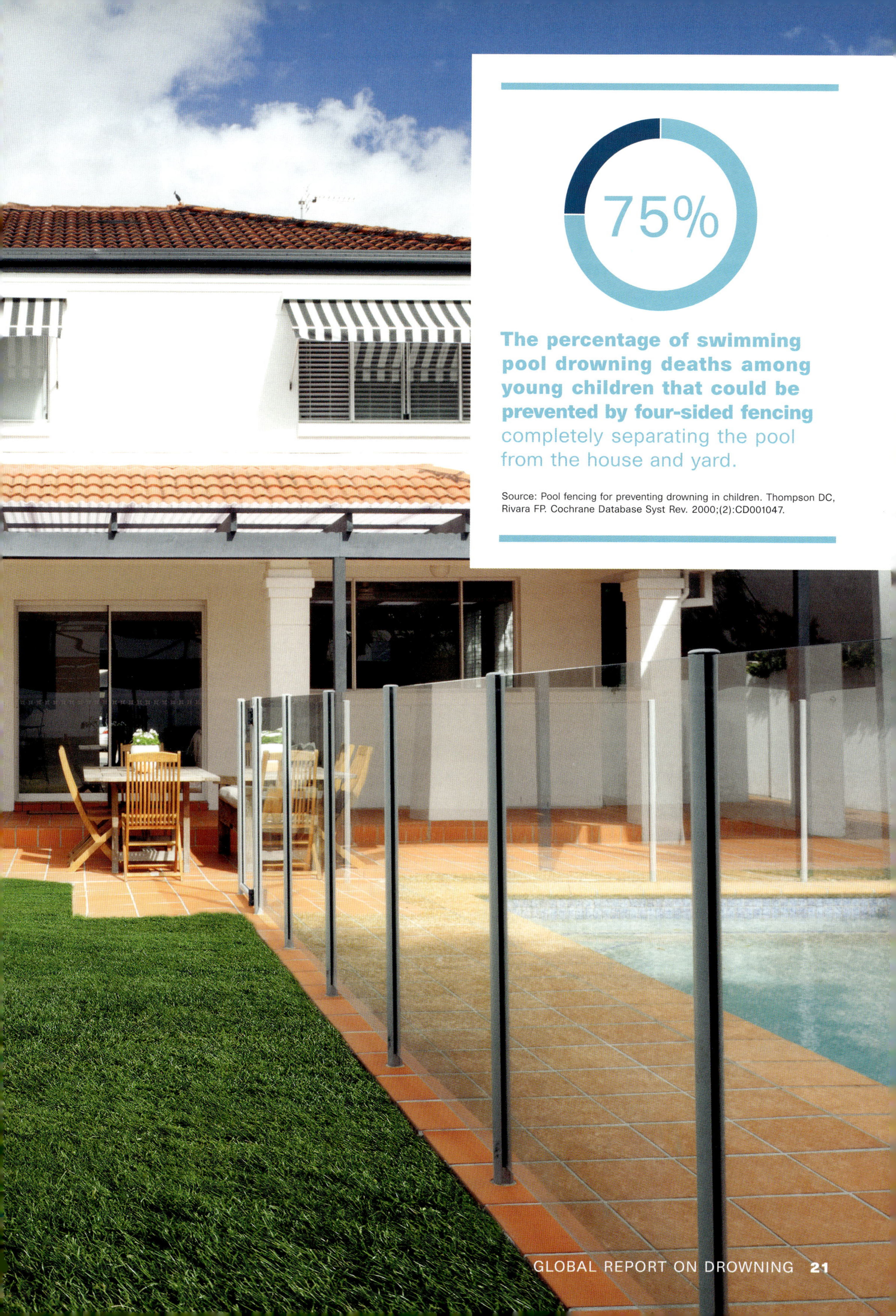

75%

The percentage of swimming pool drowning deaths among young children that could be prevented by four-sided fencing completely separating the pool from the house and yard.

Source: Pool fencing for preventing drowning in children. Thompson DC, Rivara FP. Cochrane Database Syst Rev. 2000;(2):CD001047.

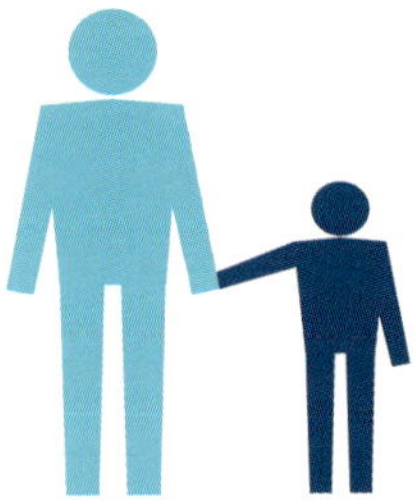

2 PROVIDE SAFE PLACES FOR PRE-SCHOOL CHILDREN WITH CAPABLE CHILD CARE

Community-based, supervised child care for pre-school children can reduce drowning risk and has other proven health benefits.

Supervised child care programmes have been established at village level in a number of low- and middle-income countries. In southern India, such programmes (known locally as *balwadis*) have been suggested by local populations as effective responses to prevent drowning associated with lapses in supervision.[14] In Cambodia, village-based child care programmes for pre-school children have also been established to prevent drowning.

A village-based child care programme studied extensively in relation to drowning prevention took place across three rural regions in Bangladesh.[15] Here, village-based child-carers were trained in child safety, supervision and early childhood development, and a maximum ratio of 25 children per supervising adult and assistant was set. Child care was made available for pre-school children from 9am–1pm - the period when drowning was most likely to occur - and included early childhood development activities and early learning, supplementary nutrition and health and hygiene awareness (such as hand washing and latrine use).

This child care programme (known locally as *anchal*) was associated with a significant reduction in drowning, and in terms of cost-effectiveness compared favourably with other child survival strategies such as oral rehydration therapy. An additional and powerful rationale for expanding village-based child care programmes such as this is that their benefits (potentially lifelong) extend to many health areas, including the well-known advantages of child care for early childhood development, and the prevention of other child injuries and infections.

Such efforts should be systematically implemented and monitored in order to identify best practices, with a particular focus on identifying how these can be brought to scale in low- and middle-income countries.

14 Isaac R et al. Community perception of child drowning in South India: a qualitative study. Annals of Tropical Paediatrics. 2007;27(3):225–229. doi:10.1179/146532807x220343.

15 Rahman F, Bose S, Linnan M et al. Cost-Effectiveness of an injury anddrowning prevention program in Bangladesh. Pediatrics. 2012 Dec;130(6):e1621–8.

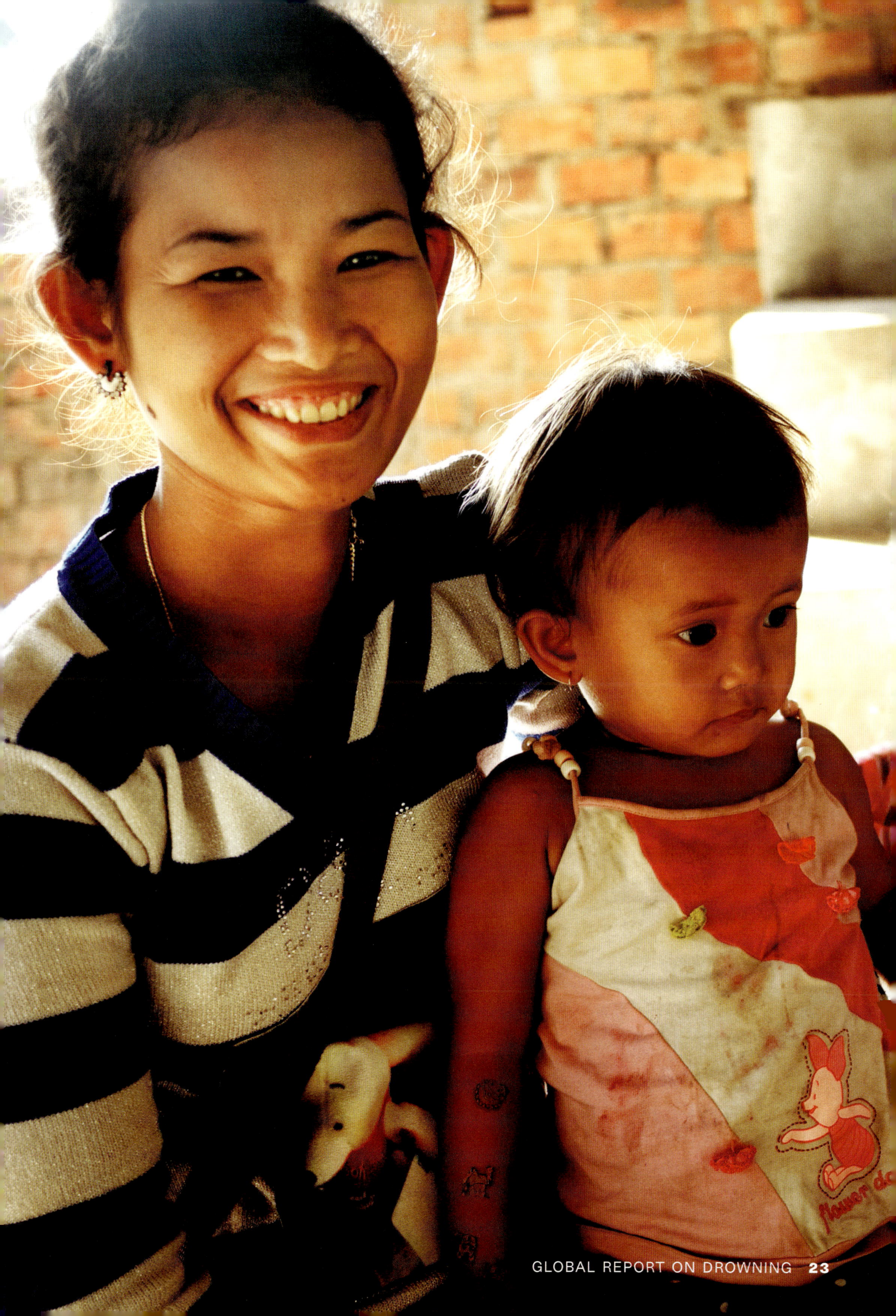

Instructor providing swim skills training in a high-income setting.

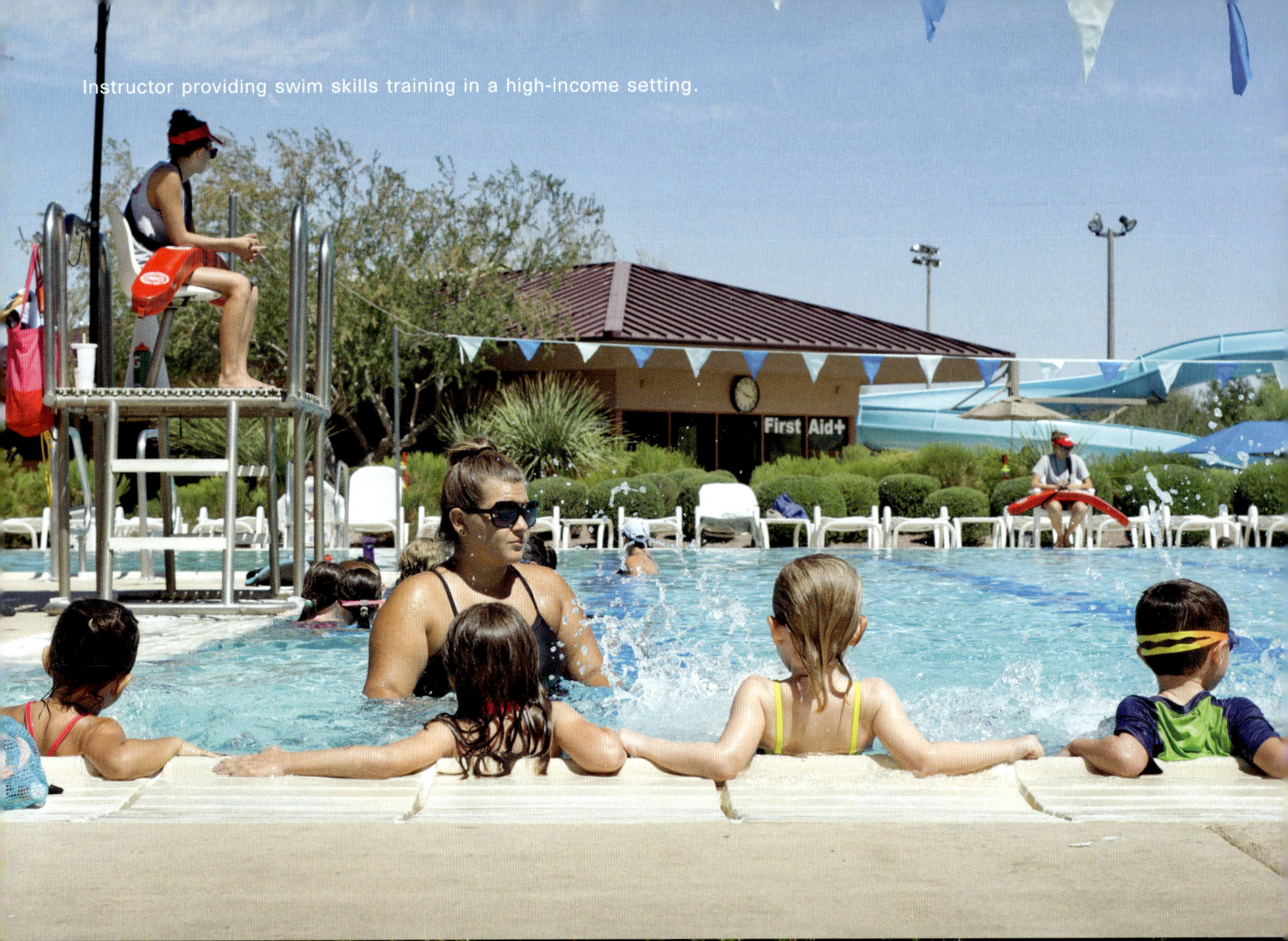

Instructor providing swim skills training in a low-income setting. A submerged platform limits the depth to 1 metre where these children are learning kicking skills. The area outside is deeper, permitting children to practice in water that may go over their heads. The training area is enclosed by bamboo fencing to limit access to the larger pond.

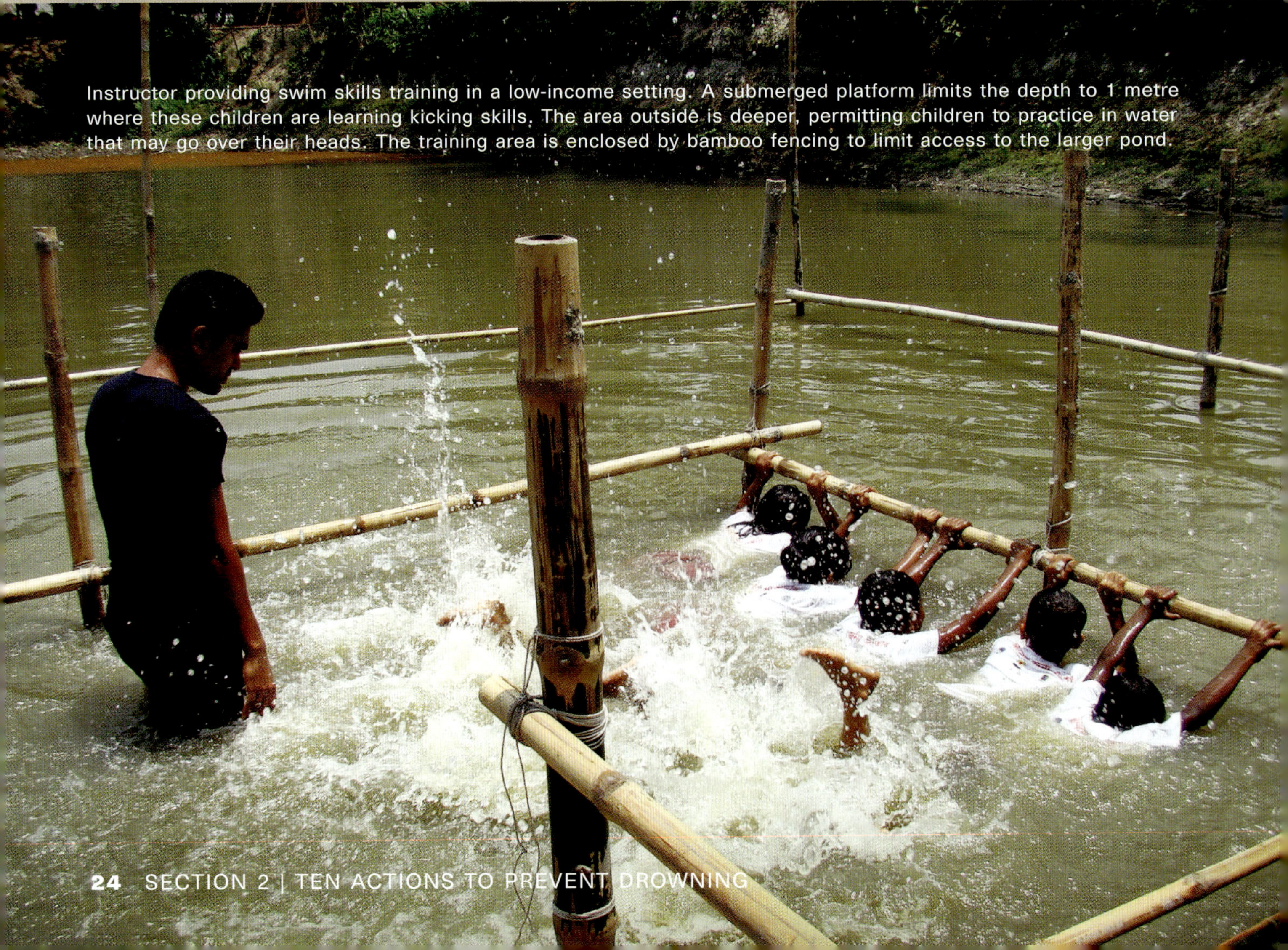

3 TEACH SCHOOL-AGE CHILDREN BASIC SWIMMING, WATER SAFETY AND SAFE RESCUE SKILLS

Studies of programmes in Australia, Bangladesh, China, Thailand, the United States and Viet Nam show that teaching children basic swimming, water safety and safe rescue skills reduces drowning. Based on this knowledge, systematic and carefully monitored replication of such programmes will help clarify best practice.

Most recently, a study was made of almost 80,000 children aged 4–12 years who completed the SwimSafe programme in Bangladesh. SwimSafe is a structured programme that requires children to learn 21 steps of swimming skills, typically over 14 days.[16] The training dramatically reduced the likelihood of drowning, and was shown to be very cost-effective under the WHO-CHOICE criteria, meaning this intervention compares very favourably with other child survival interventions.

To replicate these results in other resource-poor settings with high drowning risk, such programmes should include the following:

1. **A structured, safety-tested curriculum.** The SwimSafe curriculum[17] developed from local studies (in Bangladesh, Thailand and Viet Nam) of how children acquire swimming skills in each setting. These were then ranked for safety and effectiveness. Following this, best practices were adapted in line with established swim training curricula. These include identifying children with conditions (e.g. seizures or respiratory disorders) that may place them at increased risk of drowning during swim skills training, and ensuring these are dealt with appropriately. The objective is a safe, structured curriculum adapted to the local population and context.

2. **A safe training environment.** Physically demarcated areas in village ponds with submerged platforms or above-ground, transportable pools filled with fresh water to a controllable depth are examples of training environments adapted to local settings. These provide safe areas where children can be actively supervised while they learn.

3. **Trained instructors.** Programmes must be established in safe and controlled environments with trained instructors who are well versed in the curriculum, its training methods and what is expected of them in relation to supervision.

4. **Student-instructor ratios established for safety.** These should be appropriate for the skill level and water conditions, with due consideration for the safety of all taking part.

Underlying these prerequisites for teaching children to swim is a heavy emphasis on safety. Curricula, training environment, screening and student selection, instructors and student-instructor ratios all need to be seen as part of an overall risk management system. Training children to swim is an inherently dangerous process, and swim skills training should be approached as a public health intervention – where safety should be demonstrated and constantly monitored.

16 Rahman F, Bose S, Linnan M et al. Cost-Effectiveness of an injury and drowning prevention program in Bangladesh. Pediatrics. 2012 Dec;130(6):e1621–8.

17 See www.swimsafe.org.

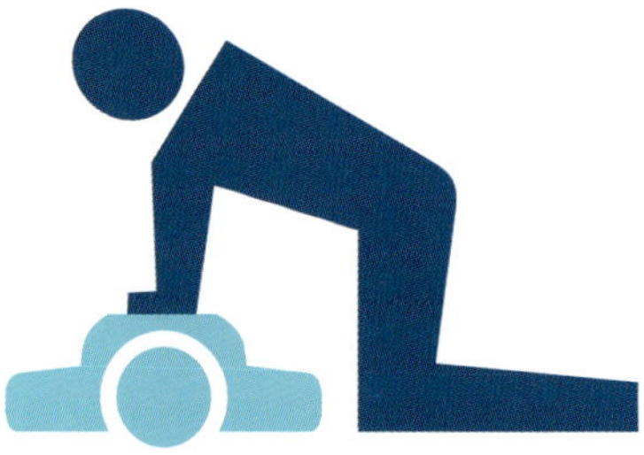

4 TRAIN BYSTANDERS IN SAFE RESCUE AND RESUSCITATION

SAFE RESCUE

Some rescue attempts end with the rescuer fatally drowning, either because they could not swim well or were not aware of simple, safe rescue techniques that avoid entering the water, such as using a rod or pole, throwing a rope, lifebuoy or improvised life-line such as a garden hose.

But rescue can be done safely, and bystanders' actions can make a critical difference.[18] Given the importance of removing the drowning person from the water immediately, and the principle that rescuers must not put themselves at risk, awareness of safe rescue techniques should be a focus of community-based awareness raising, and part of learn-to-swim programmes.

The International Life Saving Federation (ILS) provides technical guidance on how these skills should be taught and assessed, recommending that basic aquatic survival skills training includes the ability to "rescue and be rescued by extending or grasping a rescue aid (for example a pole, bottle, rope etc.) and be guided to safety over a distance (i.e. 3 to 5 metres)". Successful programmes promoting skills such as these have been carried out by the ILS and others, including (over many years) the Herald Sun programme in Victoria, Australia, Red Cross Societies in a range of countries and the YMCA programmes in the United States.

RESUSCITATION

There is strong evidence that CPR - meaning both chest compression and mouth-to-mouth resuscitation - is the only way to prevent death when a drowning victim has no pulse and is not breathing (see Box 4). Survival improves when appropriate resuscitation is performed as soon as submersion is over, although survivors may have severe neurological damage if there has been a prolonged stoppage of the heart and breathing.[19,20]

A simplified method of CPR that involves chest compressions only (i.e. no mouth-to-mouth resuscitation) has been promoted for untrained first aiders witnessing cardiac arrests, but it is important to note that this so-called hands-only CPR is not appropriate for drowning victims who have no pulse and are not breathing. An ILS statement on this issue draws attention to the role played by lack of oxygen in relation to heart stoppage caused by drowning, and a recent review has outlined more areas where the approach to CPR for drowning victims is different to that for cases of cardiac arrest.[21]

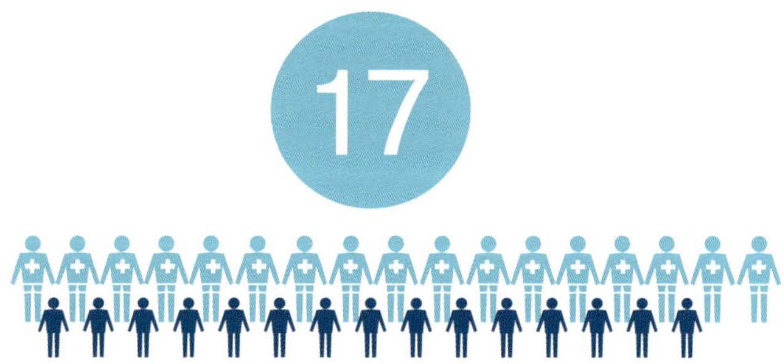

The number of rescuers fatally drowned in 15 incidents in Australia (2002–2007) trying to rescue a drowning child. In 93% of these incidents, the child survived.

Source: Franklin R, Pearn J. Drowning for love: the aquatic victim-instead-of-rescuer syndrome: drowning fatalities involving those attempting to rescue a child. Journal of Paediatrics and Child Health. 2011;47(1-2)44-7.

18 Venema A, Groothoff J, Bierens J. The role of bystanders during rescue and resuscitation of drowning victims. Resuscitation. 2010 Apr;81(4):434-9. doi: 10.1016/j.resuscitation.2010.01.005. Epub 2010 Feb 10.

19 Szpilman D, Soares M. In-water resuscitation - is it worthwhile? Resuscitation. 2004 Oct;63(1):25-31.

20 Drowning resuscitation requires another state of mind. Bierens J, Warner, DS. Resuscitation. Volume 84, Issue 11, 1467-1469.

21 Szpilman D, Bierens J, Handley A, Orlowski J. Drowning. New England Journal of Medicine. 2012;366(22):2102-2110.

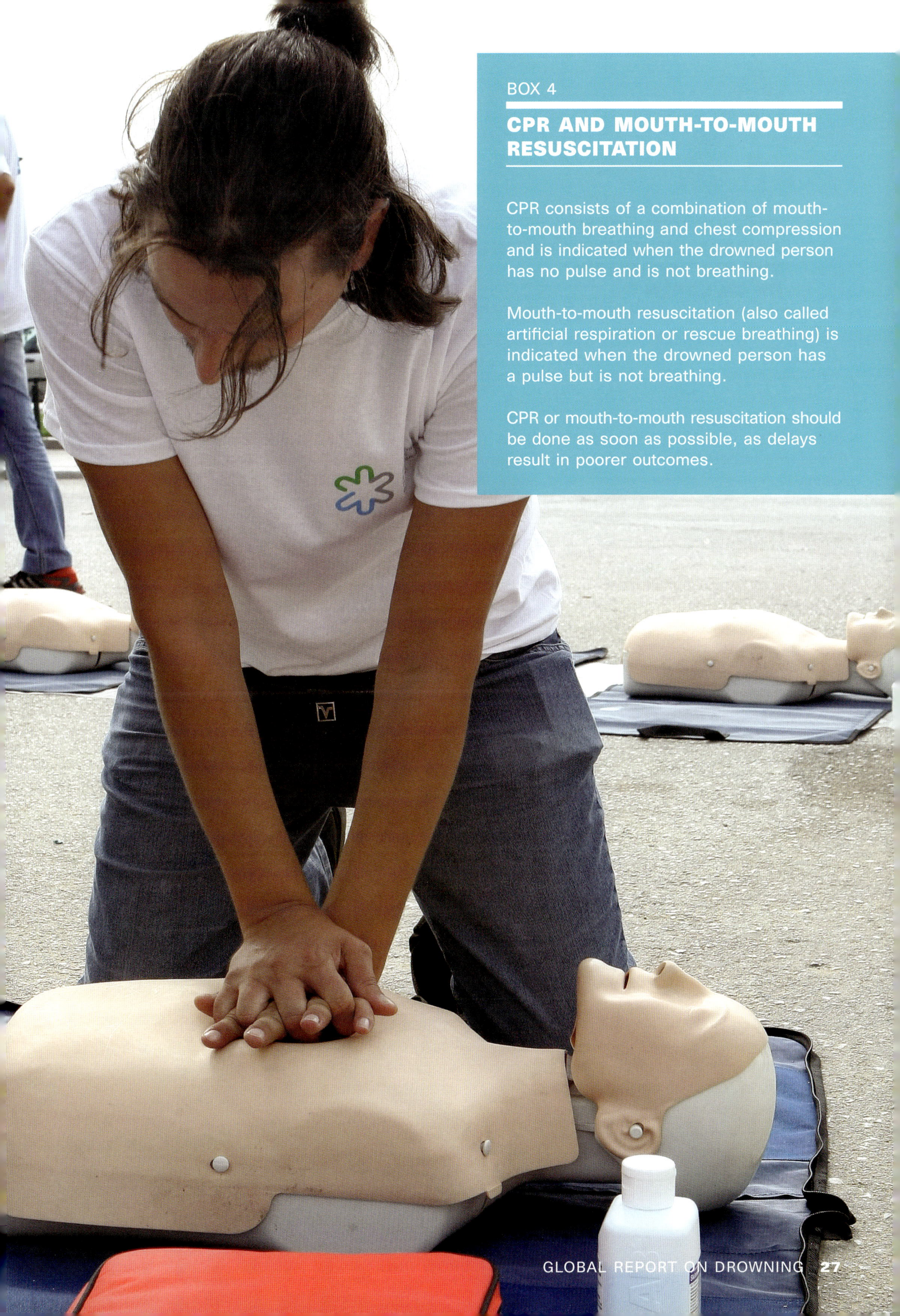

BOX 4

CPR AND MOUTH-TO-MOUTH RESUSCITATION

CPR consists of a combination of mouth-to-mouth breathing and chest compression and is indicated when the drowned person has no pulse and is not breathing.

Mouth-to-mouth resuscitation (also called artificial respiration or rescue breathing) is indicated when the drowned person has a pulse but is not breathing.

CPR or mouth-to-mouth resuscitation should be done as soon as possible, as delays result in poorer outcomes.

5 STRENGTHEN PUBLIC AWARENESS AND HIGHLIGHT THE VULNERABILITY OF CHILDREN

Governments and communities in many high-income countries and some low- and middle-income countries have made progress on drowning prevention. For those yet to gain the necessary momentum to engage with the issue in a targeted way there are many rapid gains to be had. Creating public awareness is a powerful tool for achieving this.

Public awareness is most effective when it is:

- directed at specific risk factors, such as ensuring adult supervision of young children or reducing exposure to water hazards;
- coordinated with practical interventions such as community child care, basic swimming lessons, and low-cost protective items such as well covers and playpens;
- linked to strengthened enforcement of regulations.

Lifesaving societies, injury prevention committees and other nongovernmental organizations (NGOs) can be very active in strengthening public awareness. The ILS has played a critical role in leading and supporting the work of national and international organizations (including members and non-members of the ILS) engaged in drowning prevention. In many countries Red Cross societies have played an important role. Collectively, these entities have educated communities on the dangers of, and ways to avoid, drowning. Long-term declines in drowning in a number of countries are associated with the establishment and community actions of lifesaving societies.

ENSURE RISKS TO CHILDREN ARE UNDERSTOOD AND ADDRESSED

A national water safety plan (see page 36) can enable NGOs to work with the education system to deliver water safety programmes to school-age children. Such a strategy can also support the work of advocacy organizations to ensure parents and caregivers are aware of drowning risks for children, and take preventative steps.

SIGNPOST DANGEROUS AREAS AND PRE-POSITION RESCUE EQUIPMENT

Ensuring adequate signage to draw attention to hazards such as riptides,[22] waterfalls and fast currents is another important aspect of raising public awareness of drowning risks. In addition, lifebuoys can be placed in locations where there is a known drowning risk, acting both as a visual alert for the nearby risk, and as a potential life saver. Instructions on how to deploy any lifebuoys in hazard areas should be clear and simple.

GET THE MEDIA ON BOARD

Social marketing and media training for journalists on the public health aspects of drowning greatly increase the reach and effectiveness of public awareness efforts (see Box 5). Such efforts should target the main risk factors, risk groups and prevention strategies relevant to each setting.

22 A riptide is a strong current caused by tidal flow in confined areas such as inlets that may present a hazard to swimmers and boaters.

BOX 5

'TURN AROUND, DON'T DROWN': PUBLIC AWARENESS IN TEXAS, USA

The United States' National Weather Service (NWS) reports that 80% of flood-related deaths in southern Texas result from driving through low-water crossings, walking along banks of flooded areas or playing in floodwater. More than half of flood fatalities result from automobiles being swept downstream.

To deter drivers and walkers from using flooded crossings and paths, staff at NWS launched the 'Turn around, don't drown' campaign in 2003, in partnership with the Federal Alliance for Safe Homes and the Texas Division of Emergency Management. Leaflets, posters and bumper stickers were provided and a website was developed. In May 2005 the campaign expanded across Texas. Billboards carried the flood safety message, and in the city of San Antonio, bumper stickers on police, fire and city vehicles displayed the slogan. The message was also spread through local media via public service announcements, distribution of bumper stickers by the Texas Floodplain Management Association, animated presentations and informative FLASH flood safety flash cards.

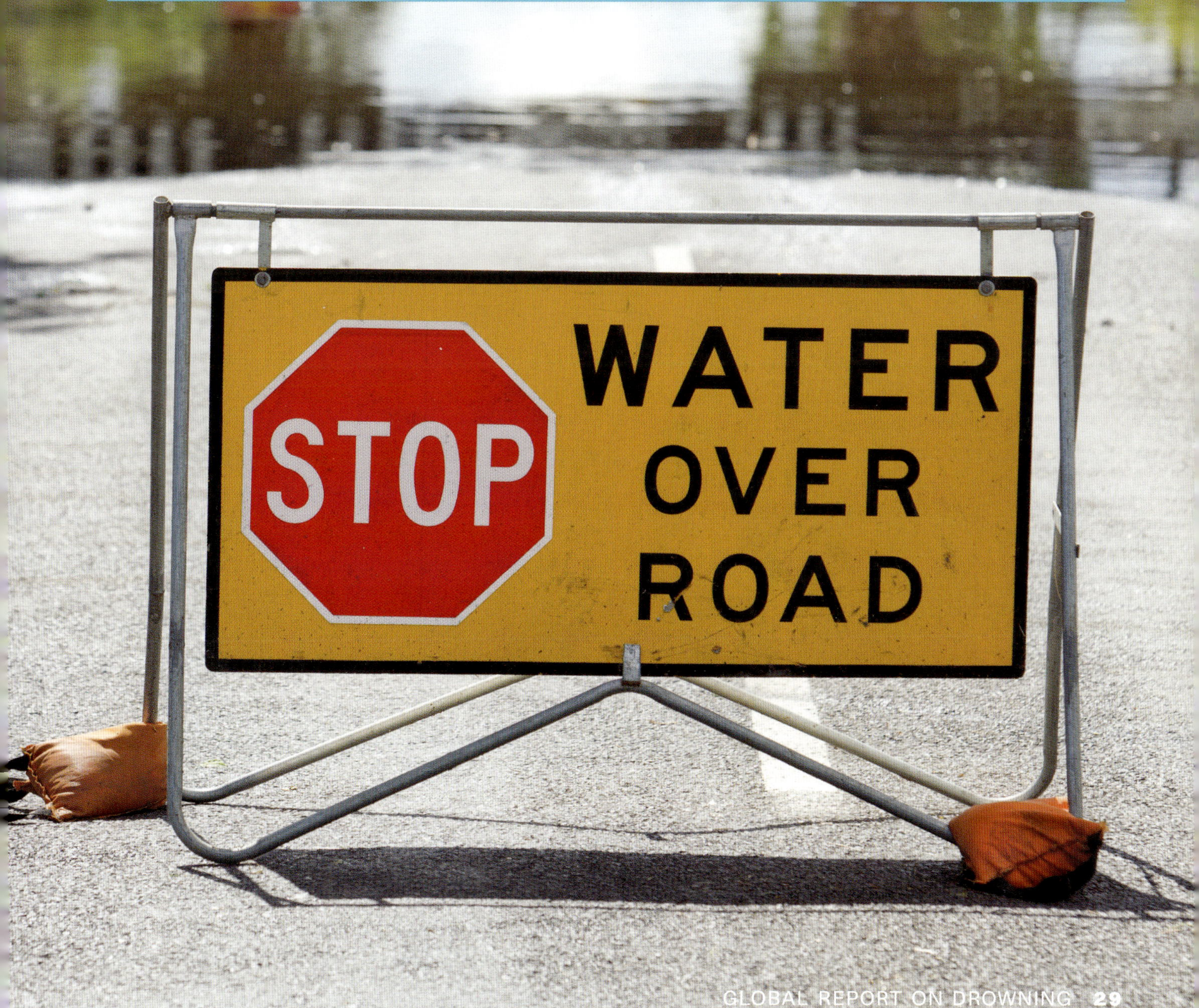

EFFECTIVE POLICIES AND LEGISLATION

6 SET AND ENFORCE SAFE BOATING, SHIPPING AND FERRY REGULATIONS

People travel on water every day using a wide range of watercraft - passenger ferries, commercial freighters and smaller recreational boats.

All water travel poses a drowning risk, but while ferry incidents often make the headlines, drowning deaths related to small boats rarely do.

Data from countries such as Australia, Canada, Germany, Finland and the United States suggest the number of deaths related to small boat[23] incidents forms a significant proportion of all drowning fatalities.

Enforcement of safety regulations for ferries and boats is therefore essential for all countries to reduce drowning deaths. Many countries have signed up to International Maritime Organization (IMO) rules (see Box 6), and base their own domestic regulations and standards on them, but their success depends on how well rules are enforced.

REGULATING PASSENGER FERRIES

Any transport incident involving a passenger ferry can result in many deaths. Ferry safety is improved by establishing systems that reliably ensure:

- the vessel is seaworthy and in good condition;
- there are enough accessible PFDs on board to meet the vessel's passenger capacity;
- the captain has the necessary skills and competence to command the vessel;
- evacuation plans are established and rehearsed by the crew;
- appropriate travel routes and rules are adhered to, avoiding the chance of collision;
- maximum capacity is well documented, and overcrowding and overloading are avoided;
- travel is restricted in poor weather and small boats are not used on the high seas.

23 There is no consistent definition of a small boat - most jurisdictions consider this to be boats up to 5-8 metres in length.

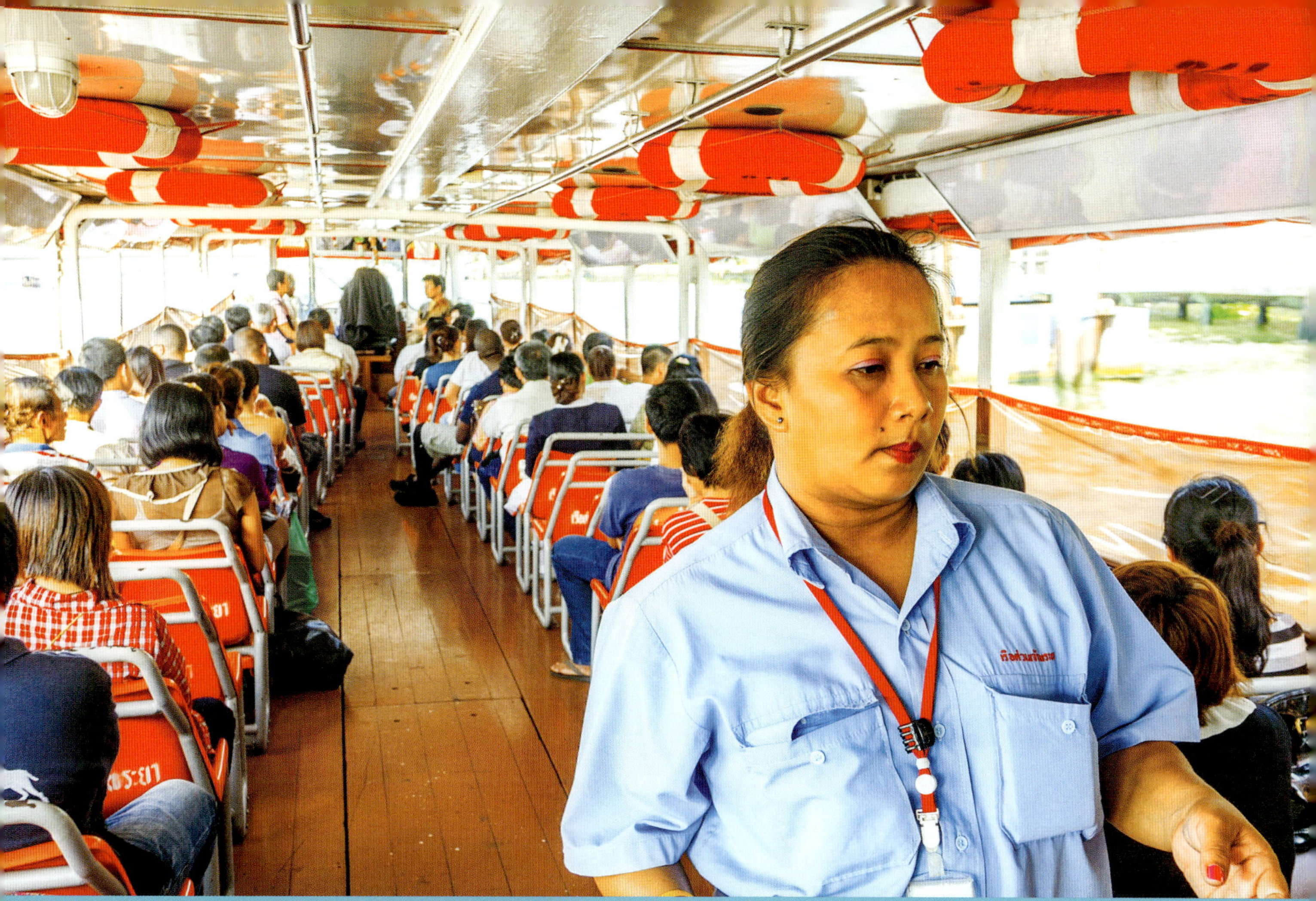

BOX 6

ACTION PLAN ADOPTED FOR EAST ASIA DOMESTIC FERRY SAFETY, 2011

Some low- and middle-income countries have adequate regulations but lack effective enforcement. The international ferry industry (Interferry) and the International Maritime Organization have partnered since 2006 to assist low- and middle-income countries to improve ferry safety with a 10-year action plan.

A detailed action plan addressing ferry safety in East Asia was agreed upon by participants in a forum organized by the International Maritime Organization in 2011. Attended by delegates from several governments as well as Interferry, the Regional Forum on Domestic Ferry Safety adopted an eight-point plan which, among other things, calls on governments to assist ship owners and operators to provide fit-for-purpose vessels that comply with national rules and regulations, and to support and monitor ships' masters and operators to ensure that safety obligations are properly met.

It also called for governments to designate relevant focal points to participate in regular dialogue with, and to share relevant data among, all those with an interest in domestic ferry safety. This will help identify critical issues that lead to incidents and casualties with a focus on formulating effective solutions.

REGULATING SMALL BOATS

The majority of deaths in incidents involving some form of watercraft occur not in transport incidents involving large vessels, but rather in fishing, recreational and small transport vessels.

Regulation of safety measures for small boats includes:

- carrying out regular maintenance of boats;
- avoiding overloading with passengers or goods;
- setting an estimated departure, return and travel route;
- setting and enforcing blood alcohol concentration limits for operators;
- ensuring boats carry:
    - approved PFDs for all on board, to be worn at all times;
    - a communication device, for example, a mobile phone, VHF radio or an emergency position indicating radio beacon;
    - a bucket with a line attached to remove water;
    - an anchor with a cable;
    - a waterproof torch or lantern;
    - a set of paddles or oars.

MULTILATERAL AND REGIONAL COOPERATION FOR SO-CALLED IRREGULAR MOVEMENTS ON WATERCRAFT

Migrants, refugees and asylum seekers looking for opportunities and sometimes safety elsewhere often take to the world's oceans and seas in what are called irregular movements - this means unauthorised travel and it frequently ends in tragedy.

The Office of the United Nations High Commissioner for Refugees (UNHCR) is due to hold a Commissioner's Dialogue on a UNHCR initiative for protection at sea in December 2014. A central objective of the dialogue and of the initiative itself is to limit loss of life in these situations. This in turn calls for greater harmonization and regulation of procedures such as maritime search and rescue (see Box 7).

BOX 7

DROWNING AND REFUGEES, ASYLUM SEEKERS AND STATELESS PEOPLE

Refugees, asylum seekers and stateless people in search of protection often use overcrowded and unsafe vessels to reach safety.

According to UNHCR, limiting the loss of life of migrants, refugees and asylum seekers who take to the sea in unseaworthy vessels calls for:

- effective national and regional search and rescue capacities;
- strengthened cooperation systems (particularly for international situations);
- policies to remove disincentives for commercial vessels to rescue those in peril;
- shared understanding of safe places where those rescued can disembark;
- possible application of approaches as laid out in the IMO's International Convention on Maritime Search and Rescue, and the International Convention on Safety of Life at Sea.

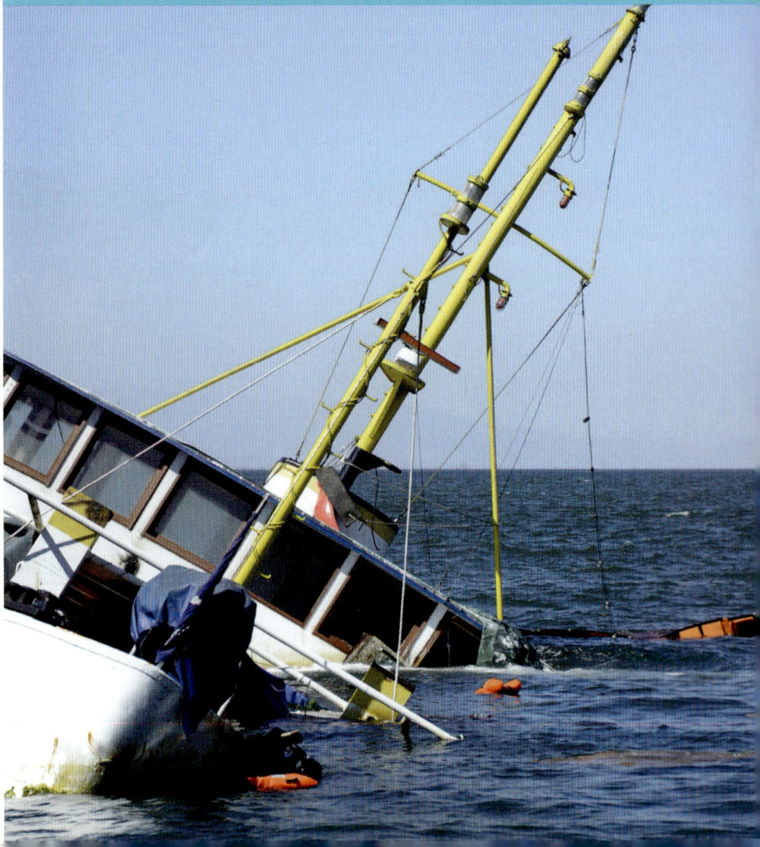

7 BUILD RESILIENCE AND MANAGE FLOOD RISKS AND OTHER HAZARDS LOCALLY AND NATIONALLY

Drowning is the leading cause of death in flood disasters and such events (see Box 8) are becoming more frequent - a trend that is projected to continue.[24]

But despite the increasing frequency of flood disasters, in some regions deaths due to sudden floods and cyclones have declined. This is thought to be the result of improvements in development conditions in low- and middle-income countries, and in early warning, disaster preparedness and response.

PREVENTING DROWNING THROUGH DISASTER RISK MANAGEMENT

Flood risk management has evolved considerably over recent years. A major policy shift has been towards integrated approaches to flood risks and the notion of living with floods, where floodplains and watersheds are restored and maintained and - for example in urban areas - flooding is managed through infrastructure such as levees, dams and canals. Rapid flooding poses the biggest drowning risk and local populations can be prepared and better protected from this risk through:

- **disaster preparedness plans with strong community awareness and education.** It is critical that local communities are involved in disaster preparedness planning, and that the plan enhances their awareness and understanding of the local flood risk reduction strategy, including what it means for them in terms of early warning, improved drainage, ecosystem management, investments in local infrastructure, insurance schemes and agricultural and land use planning.[25]
- **effective early warning systems.** These depend on a clear understanding of the at-risk population, and can prevent drowning by monitoring hazards and speedily disseminating flood warnings to vulnerable people, making sure they know what to do if a warning is issued (for example, evacuate to high ground or a designated centre).
- **land use planning.** This must ensure that shelter, housing, hospitals and other critical infrastructure are not located in flood-prone or coastal areas at risk of storm surge or tsunami, and that buildings are designed to reduce the risk of damage caused by floods. Levees separating water channels from flood plains protect against drowning in populated areas (though if damaged, they may contribute to flooding). In coastal cities such as Ho Chi Minh and Amsterdam, extensive levee systems protect against flooding but require regular maintenance.
- **preserving forests, wetlands and washlands** (land sometimes flooded by a river or stream). This helps retain natural water storage capacity, which may help prevent floods and drowning fatalities.
- **water safety awareness and basic swimming skills.** These may reduce drowning risks during floods in high-risk communities. Disaster preparedness should include raising community awareness about these skills.

Additional actions are needed to prevent drowning in floods, and further research is needed to identify the best measures to address different vulnerable populations.

24 IPCC. Managing the risks of extreme events and disasters to advance climate change adaptation. A special report of working groups I and II of the Intergovernmental Panel on Climate Change. Field CB et al, editors. Cambridge: Cambridge University Press; 2012.

25 WWAP (World Water Assessment Programme). Managing Water under Uncertainty and Risk (chapter 4): The United Nations World Water Development Report 4. Paris: UNESCO; 2012.

BOX 8

FLOOD HAZARDS ARE OF FOUR MAIN TYPES

- **Coastal floods** – including high tides and storm surge floods where water is pushed onto dry land by onshore winds, storms and cyclones.
- **Tsunamis** – where large volumes of water are displaced onto land, usually following underwater seismic activity.
- **River floods** – in a watercourse due to intense or persistent rain over large areas.
- **Flash floods** – rapid flooding of low-lying areas, at the base of hills or in dry river beds, following heavy rain or collapse of a structure withholding water, for example a dam.

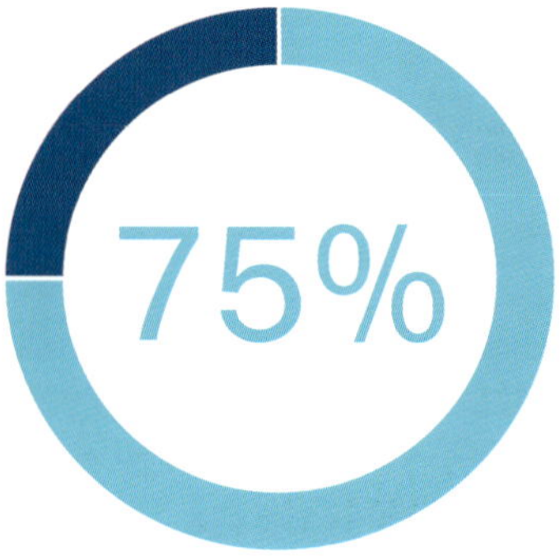

The percentage of flood deaths caused by drowning – though these are not categorized as drowning deaths in official statistics.

Source: Doocy S, Daniels A, Murray S, Kirsch TD. The human impact of floods: a historical review of events 1980–2009 and systematic literature review. PLOS Currents Disasters. 2013; Apr 16. Edition 1.

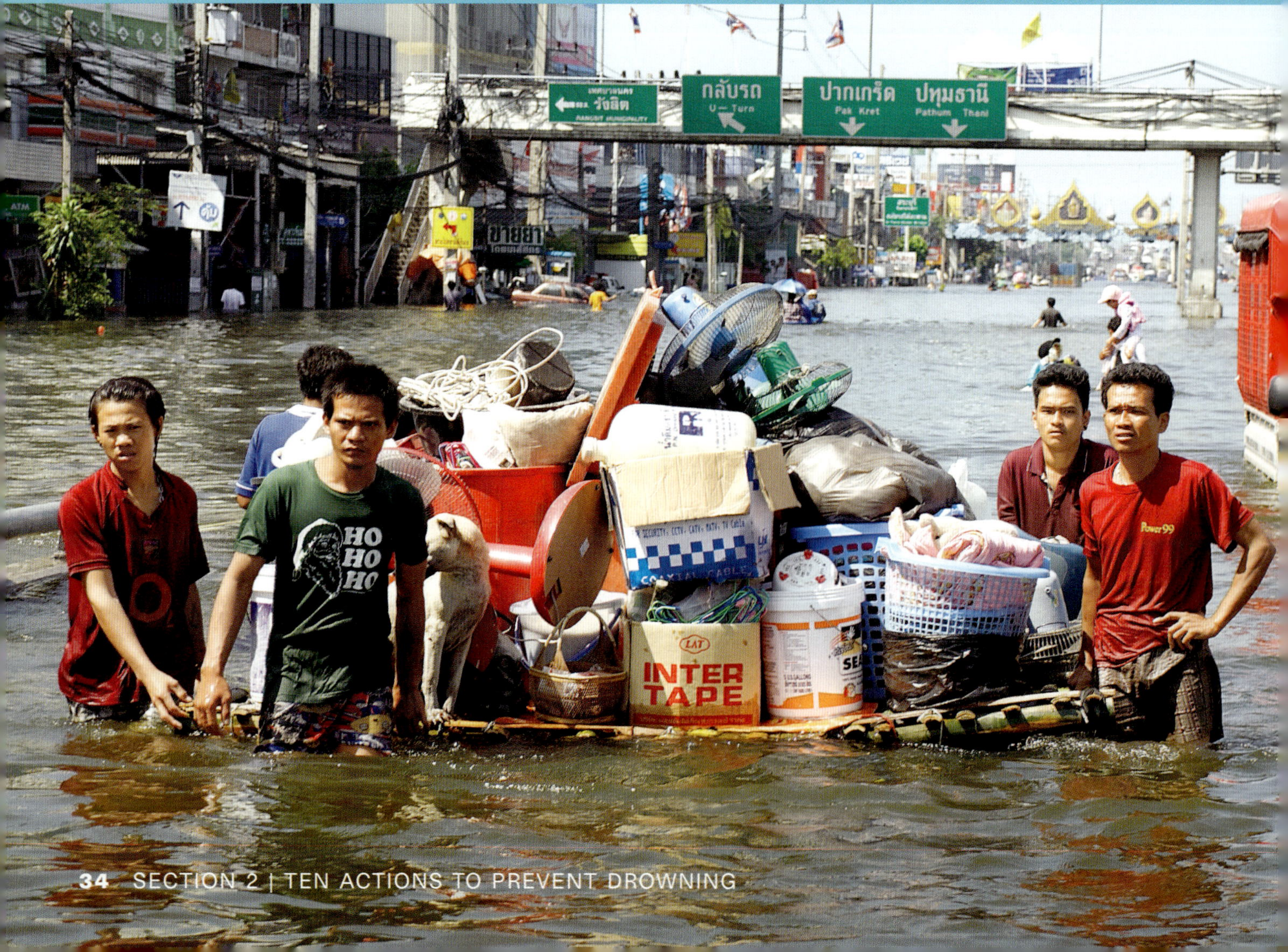

8 COORDINATE DROWNING PREVENTION EFFORTS WITH THOSE OF OTHER SECTORS AND AGENDAS

Drowning is a multisectoral issue. There is much to be gained from increased coordination and collaboration across the sectors that shape drowning risk, from fisheries to maritime transport, and from disaster risk management to health, education and rural development.

For example, a major water, sanitation and health agenda is to increase the number of people worldwide who access drinking-water from sources protected from outside contamination. An additional benefit of protected water sources – though one rarely cited in support of such programmes – is that people using them are less likely to drown in them than they are if using surface water or open wells. Similarly, controlling water-borne diseases by draining or filling in unwanted ditches, waterholes or ponds also reduces exposure to drowning risks.

Also, there are instances where the objectives of drowning prevention may benefit those of other agendas – for example, the construction of safe bridges and fords (shallow parts of rivers or streams where people can wade or drive across) reduces drowning risk, but it also improves access for transport and trade.

Development agencies support much of this work, and though they may rarely consider drowning prevention as a specific goal in its own right, they are potentially important champions for it. For example, irrigation canals designed to boost local food production by making barren land fertile can be made safe as they pass near villages by ensuring local people can cross them safely without the risk of falling in.

Drowning risks can be managed and ultimately reduced if approaches to development are more integrated (see Box 9), and take into consideration potential impacts on drowning risk.

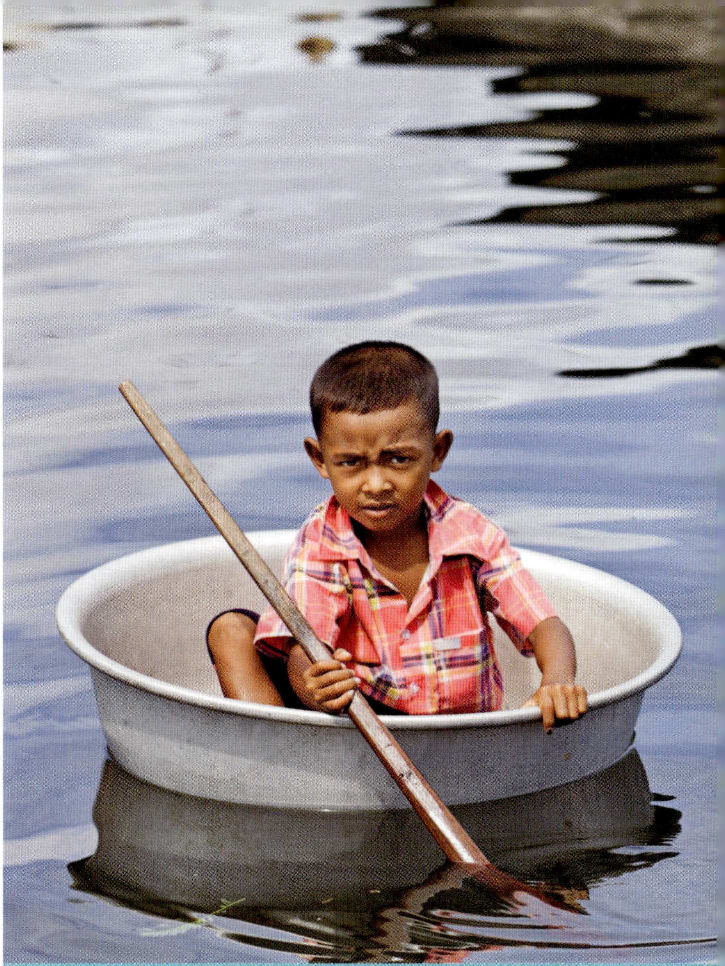

BOX 9

WORKING TOGETHER TO PREVENT DROWNING AND DISEASE, CAMBODIA

A WHO drowning prevention programme in Kampong Chhnang Province, Cambodia, targeted the population living on and around the Tonle Sap and Mekong Rivers, and who were at high risk of drowning. As this same population is also at risk of many water-borne diseases, water, sanitation and health measures were carried out alongside the drowning prevention activities to address both sets of issues.

Elements of the programme included the piloting of a day care centre run by care givers specially trained in child care, hygiene and child health; materials to build safety barriers in the homes of over 1200 families; covering water hazards; and using PFDs for small children when in boats.

In addition, the village health support group and commune council members promoted awareness of drowning in the community, and data collection on drowning in their respective communes.

9 DEVELOP A NATIONAL WATER SAFETY PLAN

All countries can benefit from a national water safety plan. Whether it is a single, unified plan or one comprising several separate plans implemented by concerned parties such as the maritime, health or fisheries sectors, or the lifesaving community itself, collaboration across sectors is essential.

There are currently a range of countries with water safety plans, including Australia (see Box 10), the Philippines and Viet Nam. There is no one-size-fits-all plan, and resources and commitment for creating such a plan will vary from country to country (not least on the basis of each country's drowning problem), but certain elements are universal: success of the plan will depend on winning stakeholders' support, clearly defining objectives and actions, and monitoring progress (see Figure 6).

Any national water safety plan should aim to:

- raise awareness of safety around water and the importance of drowning prevention;
- build consensus around solutions and develop a coherent, effective response involving all relevant partners;
- provide strategic direction and a framework to guide multisectoral efforts to prevent drowning;
- monitor action, including obtaining better data and reporting on drowning and prevention.

FIGURE 6

ESSENTIAL STEPS FOR DEVELOPING A NATIONAL WATER SAFETY PLAN

STRATEGIC PRINCIPLES

- Appropriate targets
- Coordinated and integrated
- Evidence-based
- Data driven
- Continually monitored

STEP 1 Assess the drowning situation and raise awareness. If needed, establish data collection systems ensuring data on drowning is accurate, timely and inclusive.

STEP 2 Engage stakeholders and identify leadership.

STEP 3 Agree upon a vision and principles of the stategy, and define its goals.

STEP 4 Set objectives and select evidence-based drowning prevention strategies to be implemented.

STEP 5 Establish priorities, responsibilities and coordination mechanisms and define resource needs.

STEP 6 Obtain stakeholder and government approval.

STEP 7 Implement, monitor and revise strategy and targets as necessary.

BOX 10

NATIONAL WATER SAFETY STRATEGY, AUSTRALIA

The Australian Water Safety Strategy 2012-2015 aims to halve the country's drowning deaths by 2020 by targeting three priority areas and 10 associated goals.

Supported by the Australian government, the Australian Water Safety Council* leads, facilitates and promotes the strategy (drawn up in collaboration with water safety agencies, government and other groups with an interest in preventing drowning) through its extensive community network. The strategy's priorities and goals are:

PRIORITY AREA 1
TAKING A LIFE STAGES APPROACH

1. Reduce drowning deaths in children aged 0-14 years
2. Reduce drowning deaths in young people aged 15-24 years
3. Reduce drowning deaths in people aged over 55 years

PRIORITY AREA 2
TARGETING HIGH-RISK LOCATIONS

4. Reduce drowning deaths in inland waterways
5. Reduce surf beach drowning deaths
6. Reduce drowning deaths by strengthening the aquatic industry

PRIORITY AREA 3
FOCUSING ON KEY DROWNING CHALLENGES

7. Reduce alcohol and drug-related drowning deaths
8. Reduce drowning deaths attributed to watercraft and recreational aquatic activities
9. Reduce drowning deaths in high-risk populations
10. Reduce the impact of disaster and extreme weather on drowning deaths

*Convened by Royal Life Saving Society – Australia (RLSSA); Surf Life Saving Australia (SLSA); Australian Council for Teachers of Swimming and Water Safety (AUSTSWIM); members also include the Australian Leisure Facilities Association (ALFA); Australian National Sportfishing Association; Australian Swim Coaches and Teachers Association; Divers Alert Network (DAN); Farmsafe; KidSafe; Surfing Australia; Swimming Australia.

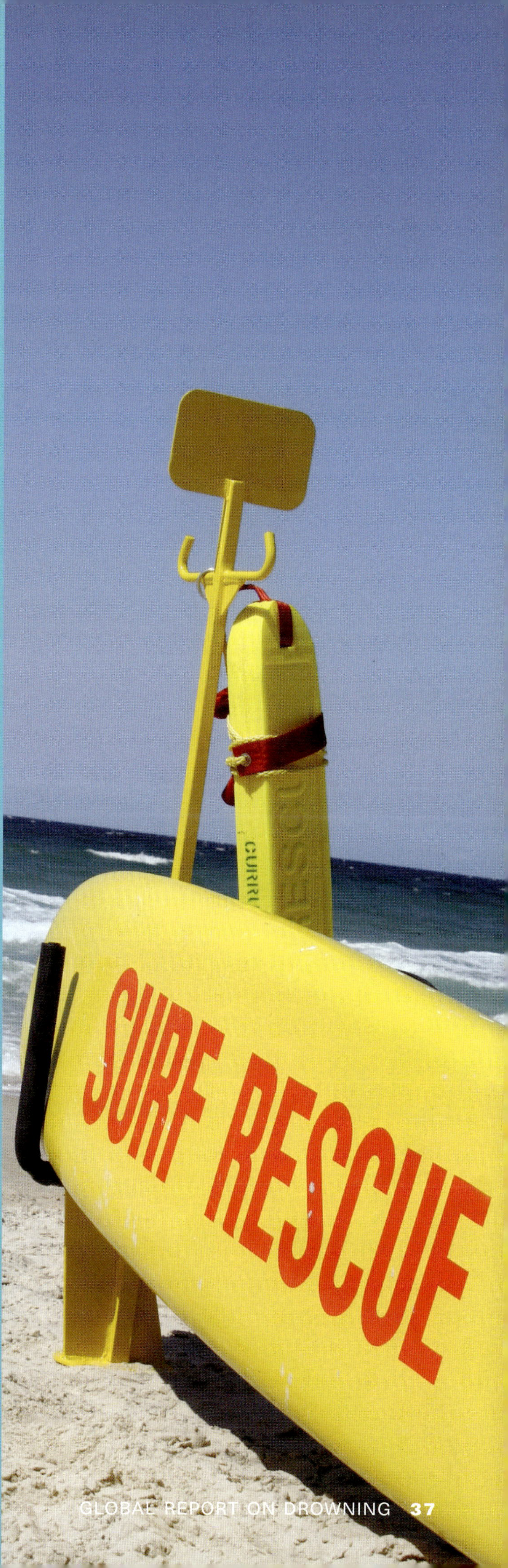

1.2 million

The number of people set to benefit from implementation research* assessing the largescale effectiveness of two childhood drowning prevention interventions (playpens and crèches) in rural Bangladesh.

*This is a study by the Johns Hopkins Bloomberg School of Public Health's International Injury Research Unit in collaboration with International Centre for Diarrhoeal Disease Research and Center for Injury Prevention and Research Bangladesh, funded by Bloomberg Philanthropies.

Source: Hyder AA, Alonge O, He S, Wadhwaniya S et al. Saving of Children's lives from Drowning in Bangladesh. American Journal of Preventive Medicine. 2014 (in press).

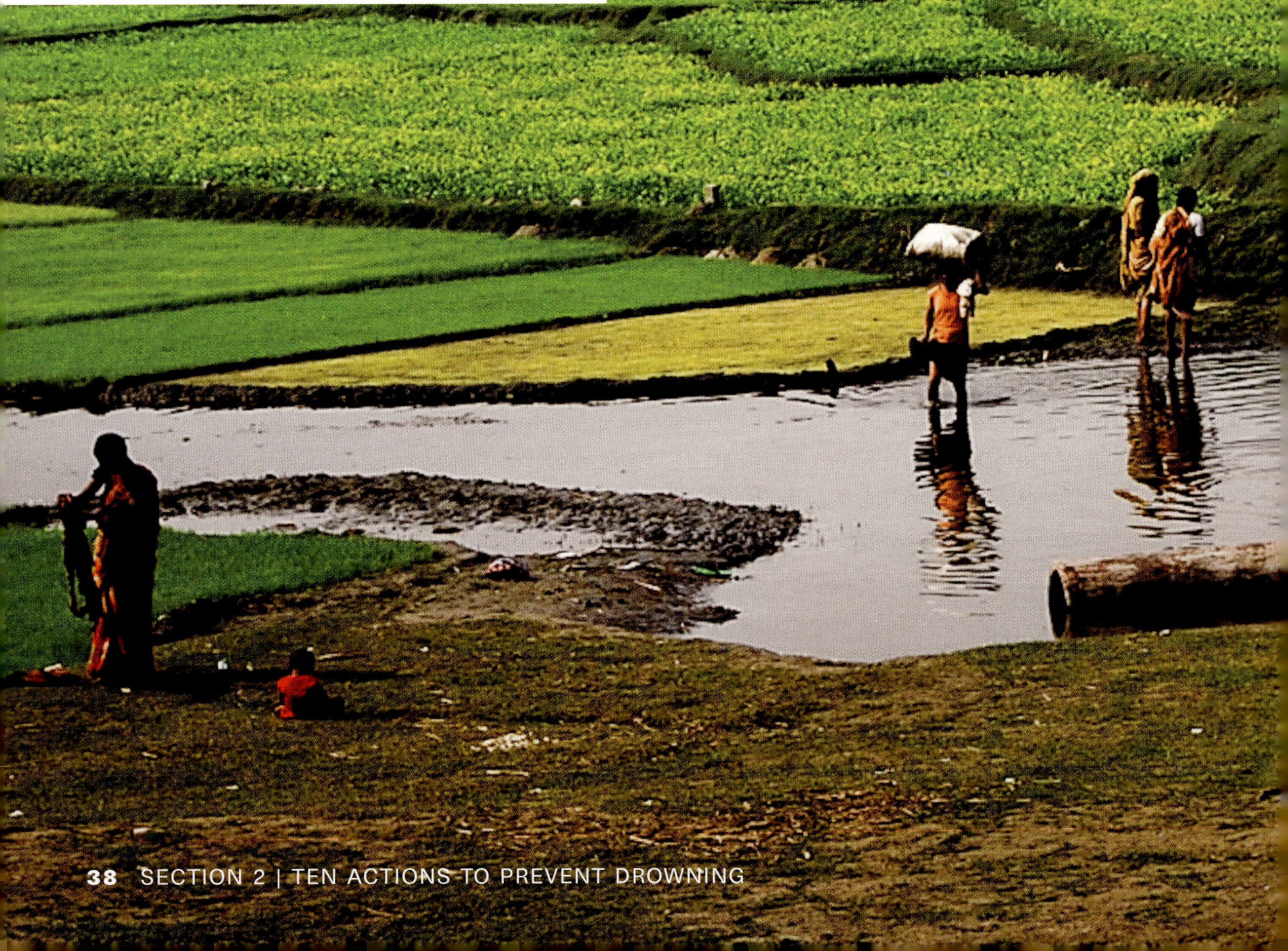

FURTHER RESEARCH

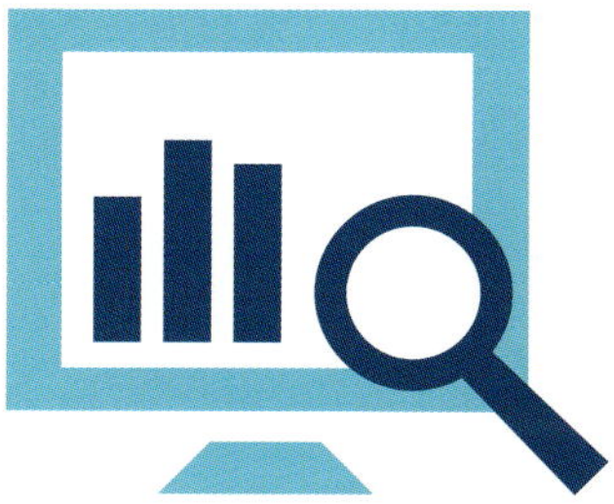

10 ADDRESS PRIORITY RESEARCH QUESTIONS WITH WELL-DESIGNED STUDIES

Further research can do much to clarify key issues and should be actively supported.

Drowning is a leading and preventable killer that has been largely overlooked, and there are a number of areas where further research is urgently needed. Key areas and potentially innovative interventions that should be on the global drowning research and development agenda include:

1. **Improving drowning data** in countries to understand the full extent and circumstances of drowning, to target interventions and evaluate their effectiveness;

2. **Improving understanding of swim skills training as a public health approach.** This includes:

   - characterizing determinants of swim skills protection across different drowning risk environments;
   - determining what types of risk management protocols - including identifying children with conditions that put them at increased risk of drowning during swim skills training - are best suited to low- and middle-income countries in order to ensure that children are safely trained;
   - determining best practices for training of trainers and identifying suitability of teachers and other community members to serve as swim skills instructors;
   - characterizing the most effective models to provide swim skills training, including through integration within primary school curricula.

3. **Improving understanding of the contextual features that impact drowning programme effectiveness,** including cultural barriers to CPR and acquisition of swimming skills, supervision of children, risk taking, enforcement of legislation and alcohol;

4. **Improved understanding of effectiveness for a number of potential interventions,** including:

   - providing PFDs to children to enhance safe access to school in high-risk locations and to people engaged in fishing or water transport;
   - establishing systems for sending text messages to mobile phones to provide early warnings of approaching cyclones, storm surges or tsunamis;
   - determining best practices in teaching safe rescue and resuscitation to potential bystander rescuers in low- and middle-income countries.

5. **Demonstrating scalability and sustainability for effective drowning prevention measures.**

Well-designed studies in these areas would do much to increase and refine our knowledge of practical solutions in locations where the burden is highest. More frequent use of cost data in the context of research involving interventions will allow for better understanding of cost-effectiveness. In turn this can help build the case for prioritizing drowning prevention, and prioritizing different drowning prevention strategies themselves. Finally, a mechanism that facilitates sharing of key findings and ideas among researchers, and prioritization of research studies will do much to ensure that resources are used effectively.

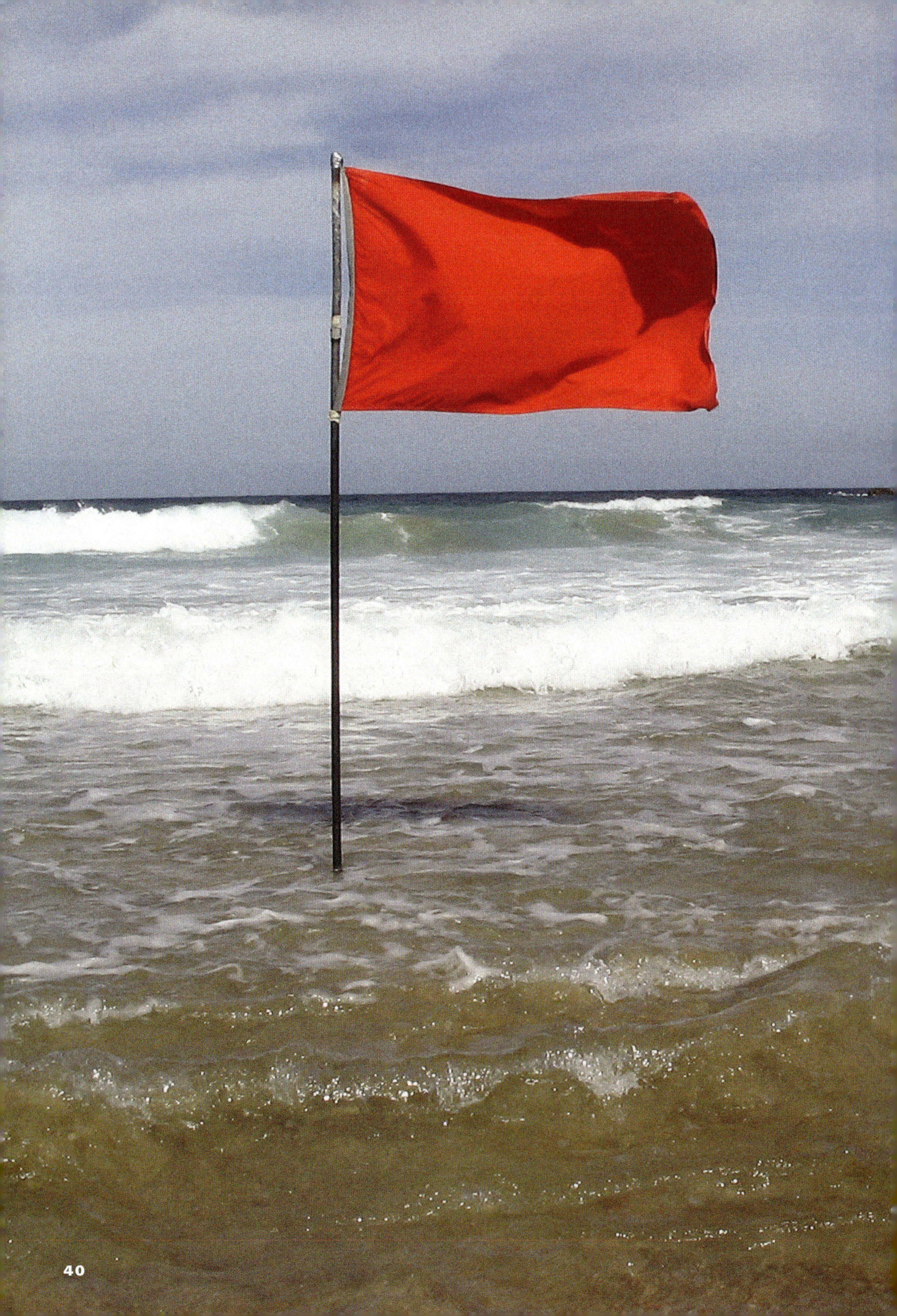

SECTION 3

CONCLUSION AND RECOMMENDATIONS

TIME TO ACT ON A PREVENTABLE KILLER

Drowning is a leading global killer, particularly among children and young adults. It is preventable but neglected relative to its impact on families, communities and livelihoods.

This report has presented the evidence for a range of proven interventions to prevent drowning that can be implemented at household, community or national level in many of the low- and middle-income settings where they are most needed.

These interventions range from teaching basic swim skills to installing barriers around water, and from providing safe spaces for children such as crèches to learning about safe rescue. Tailored to individual settings and risk groups, countries should also take steps to improve data on drowning mortality and morbidity, and establish a national water safety plan. Such plans can catalyse support and action to reduce drowning deaths, and provide a framework under which multisectoral efforts can be coordinated to carry out these actions.

DROWNING IS A MULTISECTORAL ISSUE

Drowning prevention has much in common with other public health agendas including safe water supply, rural development, disaster risk management and child health. More must be done to maximize these synergies - for example, village-based day care for pre-school children not only provides the early child development benefits associated with day care but also prevents drowning. Likewise, drowning risks could become a more clearly stated consideration of disaster risk management efforts in settings where flood disasters occur.

Given the multisectoral nature of drowning, a global partnership for drowning prevention should be established, serving as a policy and implementation leadership community for the issue of drowning prevention.

In summary, donors, development agencies, governments in high-burden drowning settings and the research and policy communities must prioritize drowning prevention and its integration with other public health agendas.

The fact that drowning has been largely overlooked to date means there are many low-hanging fruit that can provide quick gains in drowning prevention.

Now is the time to act.

RECOMMENDATIONS

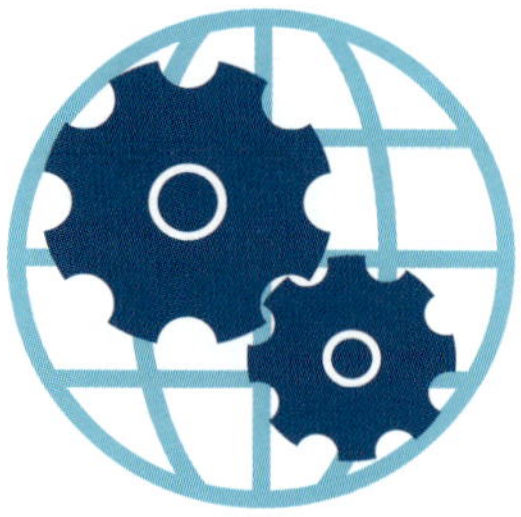

1 All countries should implement proven drowning prevention strategies, tailored to their own circumstances and risk groups

As young children are so frequently the victims of drowning, emphasis should be placed on provision of safe places for pre-school children with close, capable adult supervision, placement of barriers between children and water hazards, and teaching basic swimming, water safety and safe rescue skills to primary school children.

Governments in countries with a high drowning burden must also engage with donors, NGOs, academia and relevant UN agencies (including WHO) to ensure that progress on drowning prevention is effective and sustainable. This includes the continued search for best practices and cost-effective solutions.

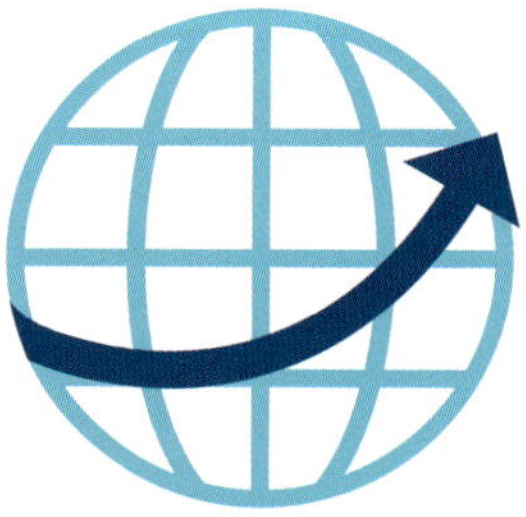

2 All countries should take steps to improve data about drowning

Drowning prevention strategies require data collection on drowning rates and the circumstances surrounding the drowning (in some countries it may be necessary to include establishing a system to collect data about the drowning of migrants, refugees and stateless people during so-called irregular travel or migration). Once interventions are implemented, data are also needed to monitor and evaluate how well strategies perform.

Countries should implement death registration and/or increase coverage to close to 100% of deaths, including in rural areas, and code deaths using International Classification of Disease (ICD-10) rules. For settings where it will take time to achieve a fully functioning vital registration system, sample vital registration using verbal autopsy in surveys and censuses can be performed. These should use the WHO verbal autopsy instrument that covers drowning. Consideration can also be given to establishing fatal injury surveillance systems in mortuaries and hospitals following WHO guidance.

3 All countries should aim to develop a national water safety plan

The plan should be broadly in line with the description of the national plan given in this report (page 36) and may draw inspiration from the national plans referenced in Appendix 1 (see pages 47-48). The national plan should also include the human and financial resources to implement it. The plan should set appropriate targets relevant to the drowning situation in each country, and outline the evidence-based mechanisms that will be used to achieve those targets.

The national plan should be developed either in a process that involves a review of legislation and standards governing water safety and boating regulations and flood disaster risk management measures, or if the strategy already exists, these issues should be reviewed as part of a regular and recurring progress review. Action should be taken to implement enforcement campaigns to ensure the safety of those working or travelling on or around water.

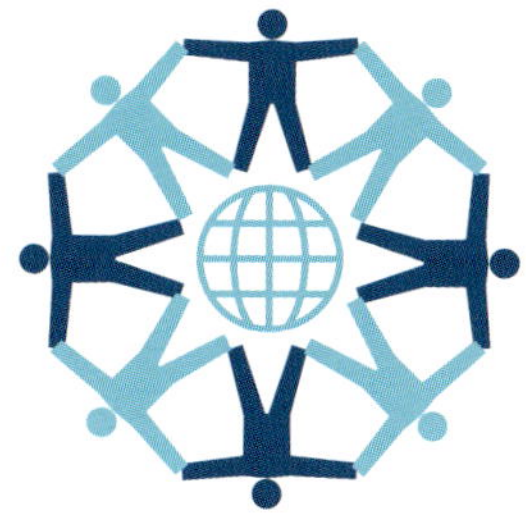

4 A global partnership for drowning prevention should be established

Given the multisectoral nature of the drowning problem and the relative lack of coordinated engagement to date on this issue, a partnership could do a great deal to catalyse and advance work on drowning prevention. The establishment of a global platform to prevent drowning has been recommended and discussed during the last two World Conferences on Drowning Prevention – a biannual conference organized by the ILS. The aim of the partnership would be to serve as a policy and implementation leadership community on drowning prevention. Objectives of the partnership would include: setting priorities for further development of the drowning prevention field; technical exchange; improvements in gathering drowning mortality and morbidity data; development of guidance for drowning prevention for governments; and raising the profile of drowning prevention in relevant political and public health discussions.

Membership of the partnership should include representation from relevant UN agencies including WHO, IMO, UNICEF and UNISDR; international federations with a focus on swimming and drowning such as ILS; key development assistance agencies; key NGOs and academic institutions engaged in drowning prevention, rural development, disaster preparedness, safe drinking water and child survival issues; public health agencies; and representation from relevant government and industry sectors of a number of core countries with a high drowning burden.

APPENDIX 1

PREVENTING DROWNING – FURTHER READING AND RESOURCES

This section provides further reading and resources on some of the drowning prevention strategies discussed in this report.

INSTALL BARRIERS CONTROLLING ACCESS TO WATER

Product safety standards for barriers are important, particularly when considering how to manufacture them at scale and how they can be used in a wide variety of settings without compromising the essential attributes specified by relevant product safety standards.

The most recent product safety standards for playpens, safety barriers and swimming pool fencing (from Australia, the USA and Europe are:

PLAYPENS

- EN 12227:2010, Playpens for domestic use - safety requirements and test methods.
- ASTM F406-13, Standard consumer safety specification for non-full-size baby cribs/ play yards.

SAFETY BARRIERS (EXPANSION GATES AND EXPANDABLE ENCLOSURES)

- EN 1930:2011, Child use and care articles - safety barriers - safety requirements and test methods.
- ASTM F1004-12, Standard consumer safety specification for expansion gates and expandable enclosures.

SWIMMING POOL FENCING

- AS 1926.1-2012, Swimming pool safety - safety barriers for swimming pools.

For more information on these standards, visit the relevant standard-issuing body:

- European Standards
  www.en-standard.eu
- AS Standard (Australia)
  www.standards.org.au
- ASTM International (USA)
  www.astm.org

PROVIDE SAFE PLACES AWAY FROM WATER FOR PRE-SCHOOL CHILDREN, WITH CAPABLE CHILD CARE

VILLAGE-BASED CRÈCHE CASE STUDY, BANGLADESH

As described in Section 2, 'Provide safe places away from water for pre-school children, with capable child care', a retrospective cohort analysis in Bangladesh followed a total of 18 596 children with access to village-based crèches for an average of 2.6 years between 2006 and 2010; these were compared to matched controls. The children who participated in the village crèche had an 82% lower chance of drowning than children who did not participate in the crèche.

For more information see Rahman F, Bose S, Linnan L, Rahman A, Mashreky S, Haaland B, Finkelstein E. Cost-effectiveness of an injury and drowning prevention program in Bangladesh. Pediatrics. 2012;130(6).

TEACH SCHOOL-AGE CHILDREN BASIC SWIMMING, WATER SAFETY AND SAFE RESCUE SKILLS

SWIMSAFE BANGLADESH CASE STUDY

SwimSafe is a basic swimming programme (using a well-defined stroke) running in Bangladesh, Thailand and Viet Nam. Section 2 provides strong evidence of the benefits of trained instructors teaching basic swimming and safe rescue to rural children aged 4–12 years in controlled environments to prevent drowning.

This 2006–2010 retrospective cohort study of 79 421 participant children and matched control groups showed a 93% reduction in fatal drowning in participants compared to those in non-attending control groups.

SwimSafe Bangladesh:

- teaches basic swimming, water safety and safe rescue skills;
- uses village ponds modified with submerged platforms for safe training;
- uses a curriculum developed locally and certified by the Royal Life Saving Society of Australia;
- includes child participants age 3–17 years;
- is free to child participants;
- implements child-to-trained instructor ratios of between 2:1 and 5:1 based on children's ability, age and other factors such as malnutrition, asthma, seizures, learning or physical disabilities;
- is usually delivered in 14 lessons over two weeks;
- has already been taught to over 400 000 children.

For more information see Rahman F, Bose S, Linnan L, Rahman A, Mashreky S, Haaland B, Finkelstein E. Cost-effectiveness of an injury and drowning prevention program in Bangladesh. Pediatrics. 2012;130(6).

TRAIN POTENTIAL BYSTANDER RESCUERS IN SAFE RESCUE AND RESUSCITATION

As emphasized in the main text of the report, once drowning begins, seconds count. Immediate and safe rescue, followed by appropriate resuscitation, are both vital to the survival of a drowning victim and their prospects for avoiding disability. Despite the challenges inherent in addressing the provision of training in low- and middle-income settings where the need is greatest, increasing the number of people capable of responding appropriately in a drowning situation is an important priority in drowning prevention.

FURTHER SAFE RESCUE AND RESUSCITATION TRAINING REFERENCES

- Turgut A, Turgut T. A study on rescuer drowning and multiple drowning incidents. Journal of Safety Research. 2012;(43)129–132.

- Pearn JH, Franklin R. Flinging the squaler. Lifeline rescues for drowning prevention. International Journal of Aquatic Research and Education. 2009;(3) 315–321.

- Borse NN, Hyder AA, Streatfield PK, Arifeen SE, Bishai D. Childhood drowning and traditional rescue measures: case study from Matlab, Bangladesh. Archives of Disease in Childhood. 2011;(96) 675–680.

- International Life Saving Federation certificates for lifesaver, lifeguard and rescue diver certification: http://www.ilsf.org/certification.

- International Life Saving Federation position statements including medical statements on resuscitation: http://www.ilsf.org/about/position-statements.

- Mecrow TS, Rahman A, Linnan M, Scarr J, Mashreky SR, Talab A, Rahman F. Children reporting rescuing other children drowning in rural Bangladesh: a descriptive study. Injury Prevention. doi:10.1136/injuryprev-2013-041015.

- The lifesaving manual for instructors: safeguarding lives in, on and near water. Royal Life Saving Society UK. August, 2011.

SET AND ENFORCE SAFE BOATING, SHIPPING AND FERRY REGULATIONS

The International Maritime Organization (IMO) is the United Nations body responsible for establishing regulations for international shipping, while Interferry is the main body representing the ferry industry worldwide. IMO and Interferry have together launched an ambitious 10-year action plan related to domestic ferry safety with a view to reducing ferry-related fatalities by 90%.

- For more information visit www.interferry.com/ferry_safety_project and www.interferry.com/about/facts.

FURTHER SAFE BOATING AND FERRY RESOURCES AND REFERENCES:

- Lawson CT, Weisbrod RE. Ferry transport: the realm of responsibility for ferry disasters in developing nations. Journal of Public Transportation. 2005;131.247.19.1.

SMALL OR RECREATIONAL BOATING REGULATION EXAMPLES:

- Victorian recreational boating safety handbook. Victoria: Transport Safety Victoria; 2012 (www.transportsafety.vic.gov.au/maritime-safety/recreational-maritime/recreational-boating-safety-handbook, accessed 29 May 2014).

BUILD RESILIENCE AND MANAGE FLOOD RISKS AND OTHER HAZARDS LOCALLY AND NATIONALLY

Emerging evidence suggests that the ability to swim may help people in sudden flooding situations such as tsunamis. This is an important aspect of drowning prevention as flood risk worldwide is increasing. World Meteorological Organization reports that the decade 2001–2010:

- was the second wettest since 1901, and 2010 was the wettest year since instrumental records began;
- floods were the most frequent extreme events;
- storm-deaths declined by 16% and flood deaths by 43%, mainly due to better early warning systems and increased preparedness, despite population increases in disaster-prone areas.

FURTHER FLOODING AND DISASTER RISK REDUCTION RESOURCES AND REFERENCES:

- World Health Organization Regional Office for Europe (WHO-EURO) and Public Health England. Floods in the WHO European Region: health effects and their prevention. Copenhagen: WHO-EURO; 2013 (http://www.euro.who.int/__data/assets/pdf_file/0020/189020/e96853.pdf, accessed 29 May 2014).
- Malilay J. Floods. In: Noji E, ed. The public health consequences of disasters. New York, Oxford University Press; 1997:287–302.
- Ahern M, Kovats S. The health impacts of floods. In: Few R, Matthies F, eds. Flood hazards and health: responding to present and future risks. London, Earthscan; 2006:28–53.
- Turgut A, Turgut T. Floods and drowning incidents by floods. World Applied Sciences Journal. 2012;16(8): 1158–1162.
- The Global Climate 2001 – 2010. A decade of climate extremes. Geneva: World Meteorological Organization; 2013 (http://library.wmo.int/pmb_ged/wmo_1119_en.pdf, accessed 29 May 2014).
- Developing Early Warning Systems: a checklist. EWC III – Third International Conference on Early Warning, Bonn, Germany 27–29 March 2006 (http://www.unisdr.org/files/608_10340.pdf, accessed 29 May 2014).
- Global Assessment Reports on disaster risk reduction. Geneva: UNISDR; 2009, 2011 and 2013.
- The United Nations World Water Development Report 4 – Managing water under uncertainty and risk. Geneva: UN; 2012.

DEVELOP A NATIONAL WATER SAFETY PLAN

There is a range of countries with national water safety plans, including Australia, Canada, New Zealand, the Philippines, the Netherlands, the UK and Viet Nam.

- The Australian Water Safety Strategy 2012–2015 aims to reduce drowning deaths by 50% by 2020, and has been developed by the Australian Water Safety Council members including Royal Life Saving Society – Australia, Surf Life Saving Australia and AUSTSWIM (www.watersafety.com.au/Portals/0/AWSC%20Stragegy%202012-15/

AWSC_Strategy2012_Brochure%20-%20 Lowres.pdf).

- The Philippines' plan has been drawn up by the Philippine Drowning Prevention Council - an NGO-led consultative forum comprising strategic water safety and related government agencies who aim to raise key drowning prevention issues with government, industry and local communities (www.philippinelifesaving.org/filecabinet/PDPPlan2010-15Primer.pdf).

- In the Netherlands, the policy environment has a strong focus on flood prevention and control. The Netherlands' National Water Management Centre in Lelystad monitors water flow in the Netherlands and coordinates the day-to-day changes necessary to keep water levels within the country at an optimal and safe level. In cases of potential flood crises, the National Coordinating Centre provides relevant information to decision makers (see www.rijkswaterstaat.nl). In addition, the Netherlands' Delta programme aims to protect the country from high water and ensure fresh water supply, and while its focus is not on drowning prevention, it is a strong example of how important preventing water-related natural hazards is for some countries (www.deltacommissaris.nl/english/).

- New Zealand's water safety plan is implemented by Water Safety New Zealand (a membership organization comprising boating, marine, fishing, swimming and recreational bodies, and coastguard and police) and aims to lower the country's drowning toll through leadership, awareness of hazards and how to stay safe around water, as well as toolkits for educators (www.watersafety.org.nz).

- The UK launched a drowning prevention strategy in 2013. The strategy is implemented by the National Water Safety Forum, which comprises six specialist advisory groups focusing on safety in relation to beaches, inland water, sea, swimming pools, and on water sports safety information and research. A coordinating group provides a direct link with the national government and the search and rescue sector. The forum's secretariat is based in the Royal Society for the Prevention of Accidents and it aims to have a strong voice with government on water safety issues (www.nationalwatersafety.org.uk).

ADDRESS PRIORITY RESEARCH QUESTIONS WITH WELL-DESIGNED STUDIES

For more on relevant research questions and a comprehensive overview of the current knowledge of drowning prevention, rescue and treatment, see Bierens J, editor. Drowning. Heidelberg: Springer Verlag; 2014.

FURTHER DROWNING PREVENTION INTERVENTION REFERENCES:

- Hyder AA, Borse N, Blum L, Khan R, El Arifeen S, Baqui AH. Childhood drowning in low- and middle-income countries: Urgent need for intervention trials. Journal of Paediatrics and Child Health. 2008; 44(4): 221-227.

- Borse N, Hyder AA, Bishai D, Baker T, Arifeen SE. Potential risk estimation drowning index for children (PREDIC): a pilot study from Matlab, Bangladesh. Accident Analysis & Prevention. 2011;43(6):1901-6.

- Brenner RA, Taneja GS, Haynie DL, Trumble AC, Qian C, Klinger RM, Klebanoff MA. Association between swimming lessons and drowning in childhood: a case-control study. Archives of Pediatric & Adolescent Medicine. 2009;Mar;163(3):203-10.

APPENDIX 2
DATA

ESTIMATED NUMBER OF DEATHS FROM DROWNING, BY SEX, AGE GROUP, WHO REGION AND INCOME LEVEL, 2012[1]

YEAR 2012

REGION		TOTAL BOTH SEXES	MALE								FEMALE							
		All ages	All ages	0-27 days	1-59 months	5-9 years	10-14 years	15-24 years	25-44 years	45 years+	All ages	0-27 days	1-59 months	5-9 years	10-14 years	15-24 years	25-44 years	45 years+
WORLD		372,441	250,353	893	37,870	29,690	19,605	42,151	51,787	68,357	122,089	630	26,614	14,779	10,138	13,763	14,776	41,389
HIGH-INCOME COUNTRIES		34,455	26,258	12	891	574	488	2,967	7,161	14,164	8,197	6	406	172	180	368	1,029	6,036
LOW- AND MIDDLE-INCOME COUNTRIES	African Region	75,468	50,650	170	10,416	8,852	5,066	11,203	9,616	5,327	24,819	101	6,813	5,643	3,011	3,447	2,679	3,126
	Region of the Americas	17,564	14,539	19	1,333	793	1,023	3,487	4,255	3,628	3,026	12	781	369	370	397	451	646
	Eastern Mediterranean Region	29,484	18,795	111	4,891	1,990	1,347	3,818	3,637	3,001	10,690	86	4,333	1,222	747	1,324	1,127	1,850
	European Region	11,121	8,781	26	964	342	317	1,116	2,729	3,286	2,340	18	617	120	126	208	388	864
	South-East Asia Region	130,149	87,782	385	13,054	11,738	6,639	13,418	18,541	24,008	42,368	271	9,749	4,611	4,068	5,858	5,185	12,625
	Western Pacific Region	73,454	42,978	170	6,308	5,378	4,694	6,047	5,698	14,683	30,476	136	3,905	2,633	1,629	2,146	3,890	16,137

ESTIMATED RATES OF DEATHS FROM DROWNING, BY SEX, AGE GROUP, WHO REGION AND INCOME LEVEL, 2012, PER 100 000 POPULATION[1,2]

YEAR 2012

REGION		TOTAL BOTH SEXES	MALE								FEMALE							
		All ages	All ages	0-27 days	1-59 months	5-9 years	10-14 years	15-24 years	25-44 years	45 years+	All ages	0-27 days	1-59 months	5-9 years	10-14 years	15-24 years	25-44 years	45 years+
WORLD		5.2	7.0	–	11.4	9.3	6.4	6.8	4.9	7.3	3.4	–	8.6	5.0	3.5	2.3	1.5	4.1
HIGH-INCOME COUNTRIES		2.3	3.8	–	2.4	1.6	1.4	3.6	3.9	5.8	0.9	–	1.2	0.5	0.5	0.5	0.6	2.1
LOW- AND MIDDLE-INCOME COUNTRIES	African Region	7.9	10.8	–	14.3	14.0	9.3	12.6	8.9	9.3	5.0	–	9.6	9.1	5.6	3.9	2.5	4.9
	Region of the Americas	3.0	5.1	–	5.1	2.9	3.7	6.7	5.0	5.4	1.0	–	3.1	1.4	1.4	0.8	0.5	0.8
	Eastern Mediterranean Region	5.0	6.4	–	14.1	6.2	4.4	6.6	4.6	6.0	3.6	–	13.2	4.0	2.6	2.4	1.4	3.6
	European Region	4.0	6.6	–	9.3	3.5	3.3	5.0	6.7	8.6	1.7	–	6.3	1.3	1.4	1.0	1.0	1.8
	South-East Asia Region	7.4	9.8	–	14.4	12.6	7.2	7.7	6.6	11.6	5.0	–	11.8	5.4	4.8	3.6	1.9	6.0
	Western Pacific Region	4.8	5.6	–	10.5	9.6	8.6	4.2	2.1	5.6	3.9	–	7.5	5.4	3.4	1.6	1.5	6.2

Source: WHO Global Health Estimates.
* Rate per 100 000 live births
– Disaggregated data on live births were not available to estimate rates by sex or region.

1 Estimates cover ICD-10 categories W65-W74, and therefore do not include drownings due to natural disasters, intentional drownings, or aquatic transport.

2 Values in the 'All ages' columns are age-standardized. The remaining values are crude death rates per 100 000 population.

DEATHS FROM DROWNING[1] AS REPORTED TO WHO BY COUNTRIES/AREAS

Statistics are presented for countries/areas where the proportion of the total deaths from all causes reported to WHO represented at least 70% of all deaths that occurred in the respective countries/areas.

Notes

a — Data from vital registration system with coverage estimated at 70–84%. Countries without the 'a' notation have vital registration systems with coverage estimated at 85% or higher.

b — Data only available for codes W65–W74

No. — Number of deaths
Rate — Number of deaths per 100 000 population
– — Not available/applicable

Rates are not computed for countries with population below 200 000. Rates in columns for both sexes combined, or for all males or all females columns, are age-standardized death rates per 100 000.

Deaths where the age and sex of the deceased were not known were proportionately redistributed across age groups and sex based on the distribution of drowning deaths in the population. The numbers of deaths have therefore been rounded to the nearest whole number. Any apparent discrepancy in the total sums is due to rounding.

COUNTRY/ AREA	YEAR	MEASURE	BOTH SEXES COMBINED	MALES								FEMALES								NOTES
				ALL	< 1	1–4	5–9	10–14	15–19	20–24	25–44	45+	ALL	< 1	1–4	5–9	10–14	15–19	20–24	25–44	45+	
Albania	2004	No.	98	67	0	3	6	8	8	12	16	14	31	0	7	4	3	2	0	8	7	a
		Rate	3.2	4.4	0.0	2.8	4.2	5.1	5.0	9.4	3.8	3.3	2.0	0.0	7.2	2.9	2.0	1.3	0.0	1.8	1.6	
Anguilla	2012	No.	1	1	0	0	0	0	0	0	0	1	0	0	0	0	0	0	0	0	0	
		Rate	–	–	–	–	–	–	–	–	–	–	–	–	–	–	–	–	–	–	–	
Antigua and Barbuda	2009	No.	5	5	1	0	0	0	2	2	0	0	0	0	0	0	0	0	0	0	0	a
		Rate	–	–	–	–	–	–	–	–	–	–	–	–	–	–	–	–	–	–	–	
Argentina	2012	No.	704	569	3	66	18	30	88	74	157	133	135	6	41	9	7	9	8	15	38	
		Rate	1.7	2.8	0.9	4.8	1.1	1.8	5.1	4.3	2.7	2.4	0.7	1.8	3.1	0.6	0.4	0.6	0.5	0.3	0.6	
Armenia	2012	No.	60	58	0	3	1	1	5	14	15	19	2	0	0	1	0	0	0	0	1	a
		Rate	1.9	3.8	0.0	3.4	1.0	1.1	4.4	9.9	3.6	4.0	0.1	0.0	0.0	1.2	0.0	0.0	0.0	0.0	0.2	
Aruba	2012	No.	7	6	0	0	1	0	0	0	1	4	1	0	0	0	0	0	0	0	1	
		Rate	–	–	–	–	–	–	–	–	–	–	–	–	–	–	–	–	–	–	–	
Australia	2011	No.	332	246	2	17	11	3	11	21	73	108	86	3	7	0	4	4	6	22	40	
		Rate	1.4	2.1	1.2	2.8	1.5	0.4	1.4	2.5	2.3	2.5	0.7	2.0	1.2	0.0	0.6	0.5	0.7	0.7	0.9	
Austria	2012	No.	155	98	0	2	3	0	2	6	21	64	57	1	1	0	0	0	1	4	50	
		Rate	1.3	1.9	0.0	1.2	1.5	0.0	0.8	2.2	1.8	3.5	0.8	2.5	0.6	0.0	0.0	0.0	0.4	0.3	2.4	
Azerbaijan	2007	No.	63	43	0	12	1	3	4	5	6	12	20	0	6	0	4	1	2	4	3	
		Rate	0.7	1.0	0.0	4.4	0.3	0.7	0.8	1.1	0.5	1.2	0.5	0.0	2.6	0.0	1.0	0.2	0.5	0.3	0.3	
Bahamas	2010	No.	20	15	0	0	0	0	1	0	6	8	5	0	3	0	0	0	0	0	2	
		Rate	5.5	8.3	0.0	0.0	0.0	0.0	6.1	0.0	10.8	16.8	3.1	0.0	29.8	0.0	0.0	0.0	0.0	0.0	3.5	

Source: WHO Mortality Database as of 30 April 2014.

1 Drowning: ICD-10 codes W65–W74, V90, V92, X71, X92 and Y21 apart from countries/areas indicated by 'b', where data were only available for codes W65–W74.

DEATHS FROM DROWNING AS REPORTED TO WHO BY COUNTRIES/AREAS CONTINUED

Notes
a Data from vital registration system with coverage estimated at 70–84%. Countries without the 'a' notation have vital registration systems with coverage estimated at 85% or higher.
b Data only available for codes W65–W74

No. Number of deaths
Rate Number of deaths per 100 000 population
– Not available/applicable

COUNTRY/AREA	YEAR	MEASURE	BOTH SEXES COMBINED	MALES									FEMALES									NOTES
				ALL	< 1	1–4	5–9	10–14	15–19	20–24	25–44	45+	ALL	< 1	1–4	5–9	10–14	15–19	20–24	25–44	45+	
Bahrain	2009	No.	20	14	1	1	2	1	0	0	6	3	6	0	2	0	0	0	1	3	0	
		Rate	1.9	2.5	11.7	2.8	4.6	2.7	0.0	0.0	1.6	2.3	1.0	0.0	5.8	0.0	0.0	0.0	2.2	1.7	0.0	
Barbados	2011	No.	7	5	0	0	0	0	1	1	1	2	2	0	0	0	0	0	0	0	2	
		Rate	2.3	3.6	0.0	0.0	0.0	0.0	9.5	9.3	2.4	4.1	1.0	0.0	0.0	0.0	0.0	0.0	0.0	0.0	3.6	
Belarus	2009	No.	837	717	1	8	21	11	40	72	261	302	120	0	5	4	9	1	3	28	70	b
		Rate	8.0	14.5	1.8	4.0	9.1	4.6	12.2	17.2	18.5	18.7	2.1	0.0	2.6	1.8	3.9	0.3	0.7	2.0	3.0	
Belgium	2010	No.	201	117	0	3	5	0	3	3	22	81	84	1	1	0	0	0	0	6	76	
		Rate	1.3	1.7	0.0	1.1	1.6	0.0	0.9	0.9	1.5	3.6	1.0	1.5	0.4	0.0	0.0	0.0	0.0	0.4	3.0	
Belize	2010	No.	28	23	0	1	3	1	1	3	8	6	5	0	2	0	1	0	0	1	1	
		Rate	10.0	17.0	0.0	6.6	16.1	5.6	6.1	19.7	18.1	26.0	3.2	0.0	13.6	0.0	5.7	0.0	0.0	2.2	4.1	
Bermuda	2010	No.	5	4	0	1	0	0	0	0	2	1	1	0	0	0	0	0	0	0	1	
		Rate	–	–	–	–	–	–	–	–	–	–	–	–	–	–	–	–	–	–	–	
Bolivia (Plurinational State of)	2003	No.	83	54	3	11	0	12	14	0	11	3	29	3	8	0	4	6	0	5	3	
		Rate	–	–	–	–	–	–	–	–	–	–	–	–	–	–	–	–	–	–	–	
Bosnia and Herzegovina	2011	No.	3	3	0	0	0	0	0	0	0	3	0	0	0	0	0	0	0	0	0	
		Rate	0.0	0.1	0.0	0.0	0.0	0.0	0.0	0.0	0.0	0.4	0.0	0.0	0.0	0.0	0.0	0.0	0.0	0.0	0.0	
Brazil	2011	No.	6487	5574	13	300	209	343	728	627	1923	1431	913	14	166	94	121	84	49	195	190	
		Rate	3.3	5.7	0.9	4.8	2.4	3.9	8.7	7.3	6.3	5.8	0.9	1.0	2.8	1.1	1.4	1.0	0.6	0.6	0.7	
British Virgin Islands	2009	No.	8	8	0	0	0	0	0	2	4	2	0	0	0	0	0	0	0	0	0	
		Rate	–	–	–	–	–	–	–	–	–	–	–	–	–	–	–	–	–	–	–	
Brunei Darussalam	2011	No.	13	11	0	2	0	0	1	2	4	2	2	0	0	0	0	0	0	1	1	
		Rate	3.2	5.3	0.0	13.0	0.0	0.0	5.2	9.2	4.8	4.8	1.0	0.0	0.0	0.0	0.0	0.0	0.0	1.3	2.6	
Bulgaria	2012	No.	142	107	0	4	2	4	4	8	24	61	35	0	1	1	2	0	1	3	27	
		Rate	1.7	2.7	0.0	2.8	1.2	2.5	2.2	3.5	2.2	3.9	0.7	0.0	0.7	0.6	1.3	0.0	0.5	0.3	1.4	
Canada	2011	No.	463	350	0	11	9	8	19	34	97	172	113	1	3	2	1	5	6	21	74	
		Rate	1.2	1.9	0.0	1.4	1.0	0.8	1.7	2.8	2.0	2.4	0.5	0.5	0.4	0.2	0.1	0.5	0.5	0.4	1.0	
Cayman Islands	2010	No.	2	2	0	0	0	0	0	0	1	1	0	0	0	0	0	0	0	0	0	
		Rate	–	–	–	–	–	–	–	–	–	–	–	–	–	–	–	–	–	–	–	

DEATHS FROM DROWNING AS REPORTED TO WHO BY COUNTRIES/AREAS CONTINUED

Notes
a Data from vital registration system with coverage estimated at 70–84%. Countries without the 'a' notation have vital registration systems with coverage estimated at 85% or higher.
b Data only available for codes W65–W74

No. Number of deaths
Rate Number of deaths per 100 000 population
– Not available/applicable

COUNTRY/ AREA	YEAR	MEASURE	BOTH SEXES COMBINED	MALES									FEMALES									NOTES
				ALL	< 1	1–4	5–9	10–14	15–19	20–24	25–44	45+	ALL	< 1	1–4	5–9	10–14	15–19	20–24	25–44	45+	
Chile	2011	No.	402	353	1	16	5	11	26	30	114	150	49	0	10	2	4	3	2	11	17	
		Rate	2.3	4.0	0.8	3.2	0.8	1.7	3.5	4.0	4.5	5.7	0.6	0.0	2.1	0.3	0.6	0.4	0.3	0.4	0.6	
Colombia	2011	No.	1127	916	11	103	64	64	142	95	251	186	211	6	65	16	19	27	15	28	34	
		Rate	2.4	4.0	2.4	5.6	2.8	2.8	6.4	4.5	3.7	3.5	0.9	1.4	3.7	0.7	0.9	1.3	0.7	0.4	0.6	
Costa Rica	2012	No.	124	110	0	4	2	7	8	21	37	31	14	0	0	0	4	0	2	4	4	
		Rate	2.5	4.4	0.0	2.7	1.0	3.4	3.7	9.0	4.9	4.8	0.6	0.0	0.0	0.0	2.0	0.0	0.9	0.6	0.6	
Croatia	2012	No.	135	87	0	0	1	2	3	7	12	62	48	0	0	0	0	1	0	4	43	
		Rate	2.3	3.3	0.0	0.0	1.0	1.8	2.4	5.3	2.1	6.9	1.2	0.0	0.0	0.0	0.0	0.8	0.0	0.7	4.0	
Cuba	2011	No.	262	247	0	5	5	11	16	21	86	102	15	0	6	1	0	1	0	1	6	
		Rate	2.2	4.1	0.0	2.1	1.5	3.1	4.2	4.9	5.0	4.8	0.3	0.0	2.7	0.3	0.0	0.3	0.0	0.1	0.3	
Cyprus	2011	No.	21	10	0	1	0	0	0	0	2	7	11	0	1	0	0	0	0	3	7	
		Rate	1.5	1.5	0.0	3.8	0.0	0.0	0.0	0.0	1.1	3.7	1.7	0.0	4.1	0.0	0.0	0.0	0.0	1.8	3.5	
Czech Republic	2012	No.	209	157	0	2	1	1	5	11	44	93	52	0	2	0	0	1	3	6	40	
		Rate	1.6	2.5	0.0	0.8	0.4	0.4	1.8	3.1	2.6	4.4	0.7	0.0	0.9	0.0	0.0	0.4	0.9	0.4	1.6	
Denmark	2012	No.	87	69	0	1	0	0	1	0	19	48	18	0	0	0	0	0	0	4	14	
		Rate	1.2	2.0	0.0	0.8	0.0	0.0	0.5	0.0	2.6	4.0	0.4	0.0	0.0	0.0	0.0	0.0	0.0	0.6	1.1	
Dominica	2011	No.	6	4	0	0	0	1	0	1	0	2	2	1	0	0	0	0	0	0	1	
		Rate	–	–	–	–	–	–	–	–	–	–	–	–	–	–	–	–	–	–	–	
Ecuador	2012	No.	583	475	3	45	18	22	69	67	140	111	108	0	33	12	10	6	6	20	21	
		Rate	3.8	6.2	1.8	6.9	2.2	2.8	9.4	9.5	6.3	6.5	1.3	0.0	5.3	1.6	1.3	0.8	0.9	0.9	1.2	
Egypt	2011	No.	1619	1343	5	169	118	184	313	209	258	87	276	10	116	32	26	24	18	25	25	
		Rate	1.8	3.1	0.5	4.6	2.8	4.7	8.2	5.2	2.3	1.0	0.6	1.1	3.3	0.8	0.7	0.7	0.5	0.2	0.3	
El Salvador	2011	No.	259	208	1	3	9	12	32	31	70	49	51	1	5	6	6	6	5	11	11	a
		Rate	4.2	7.4	1.4	1.2	2.9	3.3	8.7	10.0	9.7	8.8	1.5	1.5	2.1	2.0	1.7	1.7	1.6	1.2	1.5	
Estonia	2012	No.	54	40	0	0	0	0	1	4	11	24	14	0	1	0	1	0	0	2	10	
		Rate	3.3	5.6	0.0	0.0	0.0	0.0	2.9	8.9	6.0	10.3	1.5	0.0	3.5	0.0	3.3	0.0	0.0	1.1	3.0	
Fiji	2011	No.	55	43	0	7	2	4	3	5	6	15	12	1	2	1	0	0	0	2	5	
		Rate	6.3	9.7	0.0	19.6	4.8	10.0	7.3	13.0	4.7	15.1	2.8	12.1	6.3	2.7	0.0	0.0	0.0	1.8	5.3	

DEATHS FROM DROWNING AS REPORTED TO WHO BY COUNTRIES/AREAS CONTINUED

Notes
a Data from vital registration system with coverage estimated at 70–84%. Countries without the 'a' notation have vital registration systems with coverage estimated at 85% or higher.
b Data only available for codes W65–W74

No. Number of deaths
Rate Number of deaths per 100 000 population
– Not available/applicable

COUNTRY/ AREA	YEAR	MEASURE	BOTH SEXES COMBINED	MALES									FEMALES									NOTES
				ALL	< 1	1–4	5–9	10–14	15–19	20–24	25–44	45+	ALL	< 1	1–4	5–9	10–14	15–19	20–24	25–44	45+	
Finland	2012	No.	174	132	1	0	1	0	3	6	27	94	42	0	4	0	0	0	1	3	34	
		Rate	2.4	3.8	3.2	0.0	0.7	0.0	1.8	3.5	3.9	8.0	1.0	0.0	3.4	0.0	0.0	0.0	0.6	0.5	2.5	
France	2011	No.	1382	864	2	19	8	10	27	40	160	598	518	3	16	1	3	2	3	43	447	
		Rate	1.6	2.2	0.5	1.2	0.4	0.5	1.4	2.0	1.9	4.8	1.0	0.8	1.0	0.1	0.2	0.1	0.2	0.5	3.0	
French Guiana	2011	No.	15	13	0	3	2	3	1	0	4	0	2	0	0	1	1	0	0	0	0	
		Rate	5.5	9.7	0.0	27.4	14.6	24.3	8.8	0.0	12.9	0.0	1.4	0.0	0.0	7.6	8.3	0.0	0.0	0.0	0.0	
Georgia	2012	No.	86	63	0	0	2	8	9	7	15	21	23	2	1	1	0	0	2	6	11	
		Rate	2.0	3.0	0.0	0.0	1.6	6.5	6.0	3.8	2.4	2.8	0.9	7.4	0.9	0.9	0.0	0.0	1.1	0.9	1.1	
Germany	2012	No.	765	472	2	7	6	7	9	22	81	338	293	0	6	4	4	1	8	25	245	
		Rate	0.6	0.9	0.6	0.5	0.3	0.4	0.4	0.9	0.8	1.7	0.4	0.0	0.4	0.2	0.2	0.1	0.3	0.2	1.1	
Greece	2011	No.	409	297	0	0	4	1	4	17	59	212	112	1	1	1	0	0	3	7	99	
		Rate	2.5	3.9	0.0	0.0	1.5	0.4	1.4	5.5	3.5	9.0	1.1	1.7	0.5	0.4	0.0	0.0	1.0	0.4	3.7	
Grenada	2012	No.	3	3	0	0	0	0	0	0	0	3	0	0	0	0	0	0	0	0	0	
		Rate	–	–	–	–	–	–	–	–	–	–	–	–	–	–	–	–	–	–	–	
Guadeloupe	2011	No.	26	21	0	0	0	0	0	0	7	14	5	0	0	0	0	0	0	0	5	
		Rate	5.0	9.0	0.0	0.0	0.0	0.0	0.0	0.0	13.1	17.7	1.6	0.0	0.0	0.0	0.0	0.0	0.0	0.0	5.2	
Guatemala	2012	No.	356	307	1	21	16	16	45	48	98	62	49	1	10	8	8	2	4	12	4	
		Rate	2.6	4.9	0.5	2.3	1.5	1.7	5.4	7.0	5.9	5.9	0.6	0.5	1.1	0.8	0.8	0.3	0.6	0.6	0.4	
Guyana	2010	No.	76	66	0	5	2	4	5	2	24	24	10	0	1	1	1	0	2	4	1	a
		Rate	11.8	24.7	0.0	11.7	3.5	8.3	13.3	6.1	21.4	40.4	2.6	0.0	2.6	2.0	2.4	0.0	6.0	3.5	1.5	
Hong Kong SAR	2011	No.	65	36	0	0	1	0	3	2	6	23	29	0	0	0	1	0	0	8	20	
		Rate	0.7	0.9	0.0	0.0	0.8	0.0	1.5	1.0	0.7	1.5	0.6	0.0	0.0	0.0	0.7	0.0	0.0	0.6	1.2	
Hungary	2012	No.	222	168	0	2	0	6	10	12	44	94	54	0	1	0	3	0	1	8	41	
		Rate	1.9	3.1	0.0	1.0	0.0	2.4	3.4	3.8	3.0	5.0	0.8	0.0	0.5	0.0	1.3	0.0	0.3	0.6	1.7	
Iceland	2009	No.	8	6	0	0	0	0	0	0	4	2	2	0	0	0	0	0	0	1	1	
		Rate	2.5	3.7	0.0	0.0	0.0	0.0	0.0	0.0	8.9	3.6	1.2	0.0	0.0	0.0	0.0	0.0	0.0	2.3	1.7	
Ireland	2010	No.	112	75	0	1	0	0	4	5	19	46	37	0	0	0	0	2	1	10	24	
		Rate	2.3	3.1	0.0	0.7	0.0	0.0	2.9	3.6	2.7	6.3	1.4	0.0	0.0	0.0	0.0	1.5	0.7	1.4	3.1	

DEATHS FROM DROWNING AS REPORTED TO WHO BY COUNTRIES/AREAS CONTINUED

Notes
a Data from vital registration system with coverage estimated at 70–84%. Countries without the 'a' notation have vital registration systems with coverage estimated at 85% or higher.
b Data only available for codes W65–W74

No. Number of deaths
Rate Number of deaths per 100 000 population
– Not available/applicable

COUNTRY/AREA	YEAR	MEASURE	BOTH SEXES COMBINED	MALES									FEMALES									NOTES
				ALL	< 1	1–4	5–9	10–14	15–19	20–24	25–44	45+	ALL	< 1	1–4	5–9	10–14	15–19	20–24	25–44	45+	
Israel	2011	No.	45	38	0	2	3	3	1	3	12	14	7	0	1	1	0	0	0	2	3	
		Rate	0.6	1.0	0.0	0.6	0.8	0.9	0.3	1.0	1.1	1.3	0.2	0.0	0.3	0.3	0.0	0.0	0.0	0.2	0.2	
Italy	2010	No.	554	401	0	7	9	7	12	31	95	239	153	0	4	3	0	2	4	14	126	
		Rate	0.7	1.2	0.0	0.6	0.6	0.5	0.8	2.0	1.1	1.8	0.3	0.0	0.4	0.2	0.0	0.1	0.3	0.2	0.8	
Jamaica	2006	No.	18	14	0	0	1	2	0	2	5	4	4	0	2	0	1	0	0	1	0	a
		Rate	0.7	1.2	0.0	0.0	0.7	1.4	0.0	1.9	1.3	1.3	0.3	0.0	1.9	0.0	0.7	0.0	0.0	0.3	0.0	
Japan	2011	No.	8999	4812	8	23	19	30	43	73	335	4280	4187	1	8	6	12	16	29	166	3949	
		Rate	3.2	4.1	1.5	1.1	0.7	1.0	1.4	2.1	1.9	14.4	2.4	0.2	0.4	0.2	0.4	0.5	0.9	1.0	11.5	
Kazakhstan	2012	No.	872	735	2	44	41	30	62	83	290	182	137	0	23	8	12	12	8	38	35	b
		Rate	5.1	8.9	1.0	6.2	6.0	5.3	9.2	10.3	11.7	9.3	1.6	0.0	3.4	1.2	2.2	1.9	1.0	1.5	1.4	
Kiribati	2001	No.	0	0	0	0	0	0	0	0	0	0	0	0	0	0	0	0	0	0	0	a
		Rate	–	–	–	–	–	–	–	–	–	–	–	–	–	–	–	–	–	–	–	
Kuwait	2011	No.	18	14	0	2	0	1	0	0	7	4	4	0	2	1	0	0	1	0	0	
		Rate	0.6	0.9	0.0	1.6	0.0	0.9	0.0	0.0	0.6	1.0	0.3	0.0	1.7	0.8	0.0	0.0	0.7	0.0	0.0	
Kyrgyzstan	2010	No.	358	265	3	45	14	8	15	24	96	60	93	2	31	6	6	8	4	17	19	
		Rate	6.7	10.3	4.2	18.7	5.4	3.0	5.0	8.0	12.7	12.1	3.3	3.0	13.4	2.4	2.3	2.8	1.3	2.2	3.2	
Latvia	2012	No.	148	116	0	1	1	0	6	2	38	68	32	0	1	1	0	1	0	7	22	
		Rate	6.0	10.4	0.0	2.2	1.9	0.0	10.7	2.7	13.3	18.3	2.3	0.0	2.3	2.0	0.0	1.9	0.0	2.5	3.9	
Lithuania	2012	No.	291	222	0	3	2	4	8	9	65	131	69	0	1	2	0	2	1	10	53	
		Rate	8.1	13.8	0.0	4.6	2.7	5.2	8.1	7.5	14.9	25.9	3.1	0.0	1.6	2.8	0.0	2.1	0.9	2.2	7.0	
Luxembourg	2012	No.	2	1	0	0	0	0	0	0	0	1	1	0	0	0	0	0	0	0	1	
		Rate	0.3	0.3	0.0	0.0	0.0	0.0	0.0	0.0	0.0	1.0	0.3	0.0	0.0	0.0	0.0	0.0	0.0	0.0	0.9	
Maldives	2011	No.	14	9	0	1	0	1	1	0	2	4	5	0	0	0	1	3	0	1	0	
		Rate	4.5	6.1	0.0	7.3	0.0	5.9	5.3	0.0	4.2	13.2	2.6	0.0	0.0	0.0	6.2	17.0	0.0	2.0	0.0	
Malta	2011	No.	9	7	0	0	0	0	0	1	2	4	2	0	0	0	0	0	0	0	2	
		Rate	1.6	2.7	0.0	0.0	0.0	0.0	0.0	6.7	3.4	4.4	0.6	0.0	0.0	0.0	0.0	0.0	0.0	0.0	2.0	
Martinique	2011	No.	17	15	0	0	0	0	0	1	6	8	2	0	0	0	0	0	0	1	1	
		Rate	4.0	8.2	0.0	0.0	0.0	0.0	0.0	7.7	14.6	10.3	0.6	0.0	0.0	0.0	0.0	0.0	0.0	1.8	1.0	

DEATHS FROM DROWNING AS REPORTED TO WHO BY COUNTRIES/AREAS CONTINUED

Notes
a Data from vital registration system with coverage estimated at 70–84%. Countries without the 'a' notation have vital registration systems with coverage estimated at 85% or higher.
b Data only available for codes W65–W74

No. Number of deaths
Rate Number of deaths per 100 000 population
– Not available/applicable

COUNTRY/ AREA	YEAR	MEASURE	BOTH SEXES COMBINED	MALES								FEMALES								NOTES
				ALL	< 1	1–4	5–9	10–14	15–19	20–24	25–44	45+	ALL	< 1	1–4	5–9	10–14	15–19	20–24	25–44	45+	
Mauritius	2012	No.	42	39	0	0	0	1	3	5	14	16	3	0	0	0	0	0	0	1	2	
		Rate	3.1	5.9	0.0	0.0	0.0	2.1	5.9	9.7	7.3	8.2	0.4	0.0	0.0	0.0	0.0	0.0	0.0	0.5	0.9	
Mayotte	2011	No.	0	0	0	0	0	0	0	0	0	0	0	0	0	0	0	0	0	0	0	
		Rate	0.0	0.0	0.0	0.0	0.0	0.0	0.0	0.0	0.0	0.0	0.0	0.0	0.0	0.0	0.0	0.0	0.0	0.0	0.0	
Mexico	2012	No.	2479	2107	22	182	78	110	289	277	633	517	372	16	106	29	31	42	22	68	57	
		Rate	2.1	3.7	1.9	3.9	1.3	1.8	4.9	5.3	3.7	4.2	0.6	1.5	2.4	0.5	0.5	0.7	0.4	0.4	0.4	
Montenegro	2009	No.	7	4	0	0	1	0	0	0	1	2	3	0	0	0	0	0	0	1	2	
		Rate	1.1	1.3	0.0	0.0	5.1	0.0	0.0	0.0	1.2	1.8	0.8	0.0	0.0	0.0	0.0	0.0	0.0	1.2	1.6	
Montserrat	2011	No.	1	1	0	0	1	0	0	0	0	0	0	0	0	0	0	0	0	0	0	
		Rate	–	–	–	–	–	–	–	–	–	–	–	–	–	–	–	–	–	–	–	
Netherlands	2012	No.	215	140	0	6	2	2	2	5	20	103	75	0	2	0	0	3	1	6	63	
		Rate	1.0	1.3	0.0	1.6	0.4	0.4	0.4	1.0	0.9	2.9	0.6	0.0	0.6	0.0	0.0	0.6	0.2	0.3	1.6	
Netherlands Antilles	2000	No.	2	1	0	0	0	0	1	0	0	0	1	0	0	0	0	0	0	0	1	
		Rate	–	–	–	–	–	–	–	–	–	–	–	–	–	–	–	–	–	–	–	
New Zealand	2010	No.	75	55	0	3	0	2	10	6	11	23	20	1	1	0	1	3	0	3	11	
		Rate	1.6	2.4	0.0	2.4	0.0	1.3	6.0	3.7	1.9	2.9	0.8	3.2	0.8	0.0	0.7	1.9	0.0	0.5	1.3	
Norway	2012	No.	89	62	0	0	0	1	4	1	13	43	27	0	1	0	0	2	0	5	19	
		Rate	1.4	2.0	0.0	0.0	0.0	0.6	2.4	0.6	1.9	4.3	0.9	0.0	0.8	0.0	0.0	1.3	0.0	0.8	1.8	
Oman	2010	No.	41	32	0	8	2	1	6	5	9	1	9	0	3	0	2	2	0	0	2	a
		Rate	1.4	1.8	0.0	6.9	1.9	0.9	4.0	2.1	1.3	0.6	0.8	0.0	2.7	0.0	1.7	1.5	0.0	0.0	1.4	
Panama	2011	No.	143	117	0	10	6	6	16	11	34	34	26	1	4	5	6	1	1	4	4	
		Rate	3.8	6.3	0.0	6.6	3.2	3.3	9.5	6.9	6.0	7.6	1.4	2.8	2.8	2.8	3.5	0.6	0.6	0.7	0.9	
Paraguay	2011	No.	148	132	0	11	3	16	21	16	38	26	16	0	5	1	3	2	1	3	1	a
		Rate	2.2	4.0	0.0	3.7	0.8	4.5	6.1	5.0	4.3	4.1	0.4	0.0	1.7	0.3	0.9	0.6	0.3	0.3	0.2	
Philippines	2008	No.	3830	2788	20	303	280	227	241	239	813	665	1042	11	200	161	139	84	43	157	247	
		Rate	4.6	6.9	1.8	6.5	4.9	4.3	5.0	5.5	6.7	9.0	2.4	1.0	4.5	3.0	2.8	1.8	1.0	1.3	3.0	
Poland	2012	No.	1059	880	0	8	4	18	55	73	267	455	179	2	2	0	3	5	3	32	132	
		Rate	2.4	4.2	0.0	1.0	0.4	1.9	4.7	5.2	4.5	6.4	0.7	1.0	0.3	0.0	0.3	0.4	0.2	0.6	1.5	

DEATHS FROM DROWNING AS REPORTED TO WHO BY COUNTRIES/AREAS CONTINUED

Notes

a Data from vital registration system with coverage estimated at 70–84%. Countries without the 'a' notation have vital registration systems with coverage estimated at 85% or higher.

b Data only available for codes W65–W74

No. Number of deaths

Rate Number of deaths per 100 000 population

– Not available/applicable

COUNTRY/ AREA	YEAR	MEASURE	BOTH SEXES COMBINED	MALES								FEMALES								NOTES
				ALL	< 1	1–4	5–9	10–14	15–19	20–24	25–44	45+	ALL	< 1	1–4	5–9	10–14	15–19	20–24	25–44	45+	
Portugal	2012	No.	140	94	0	5	0	2	4	1	19	63	46	0	1	1	2	0	1	2	39	
		Rate	1.0	1.5	0.0	2.4	0.0	0.7	1.5	0.3	1.2	2.9	0.5	0.0	0.5	0.4	0.8	0.0	0.4	0.1	1.5	
Puerto Rico	2010	No.	29	26	0	1	1	0	1	6	6	11	3	0	0	0	0	0	1	1	1	
		Rate	0.8	1.4	0.0	1.0	0.8	0.0	0.7	4.2	1.2	1.8	0.2	0.0	0.0	0.0	0.0	0.0	0.7	0.2	0.1	
Qatar	2011	No.	22	20	0	3	1	1	0	4	8	3	2	0	1	0	0	0	1	0	0	a
		Rate	1.2	1.7	0.0	7.8	2.2	2.6	0.0	2.5	0.9	1.4	0.4	0.0	2.8	0.0	0.0	0.0	2.4	0.0	0.0	
Republic of Korea	2012	No.	1518	1142	2	5	16	23	41	62	337	656	376	1	3	8	2	1	8	78	275	
		Rate	2.6	4.1	0.8	0.5	1.4	1.5	2.3	3.6	4.3	7.2	1.2	0.4	0.3	0.7	0.1	0.1	0.5	1.0	2.7	
Republic of Moldova	2012	No.	235	196	0	3	7	14	16	16	50	90	39	0	3	3	0	1	2	7	23	
		Rate	6.4	11.1	0.0	3.7	7.3	14.0	12.2	9.4	9.0	16.1	2.0	0.0	4.0	3.3	0.0	0.8	1.2	1.3	3.2	
Reunion	2011	No.	19	14	0	0	0	1	1	0	5	7	5	0	2	0	0	0	0	0	3	
		Rate	2.2	3.4	0.0	0.0	0.0	2.8	2.8	0.0	4.3	5.8	1.1	0.0	6.9	0.0	0.0	0.0	0.0	0.0	2.2	
Rodrigues	2012	No.	2	2	0	0	0	0	0	0	1	1	0	0	0	0	0	0	0	0	0	
		Rate	–	–	–	–	–	–	–	–	–	–	–	–	–	–	–	–	–	–	–	
Romania	2012	No.	688	557	1	12	11	31	38	40	139	285	131	1	6	6	10	4	7	17	80	
		Rate	3.1	5.1	1.0	2.7	2.0	5.6	6.6	5.1	3.9	7.5	1.1	1.1	1.5	1.2	1.9	0.7	0.9	0.5	1.7	
Russian Federation	2010	No.	11981	10156	11	136	219	192	404	827	4126	4241	1825	7	76	68	92	80	103	605	793	b
		Rate	7.8	13.9	1.3	4.1	6.1	5.8	9.0	13.1	19.9	17.8	2.4	0.9	2.4	2.0	2.9	1.9	1.7	2.8	2.3	
Saint Kitts and Nevis	2011	No.	3	2	0	0	1	0	0	0	1	0	1	0	0	0	0	0	1	0	0	
		Rate	–	–	–	–	–	–	–	–	–	–	–	–	–	–	–	–	–	–	–	
Saint Lucia	2012	No.	11	9	0	0	1	1	0	0	1	6	2	1	0	0	0	0	0	1	0	
		Rate	–	–	–	–	–	–	–	–	–	–	–	–	–	–	–	–	–	–	–	
Saint Pierre and Miquelon	2010	No.	0	0	0	0	0	0	0	0	0	0	0	0	0	0	0	0	0	0	0	
		Rate	–	–	–	–	–	–	–	–	–	–	–	–	–	–	–	–	–	–	–	
Saint Vincent and Grenadines	2012	No.	4	4	0	0	0	0	0	1	0	3	0	0	0	0	0	0	0	0	0	
		Rate	–	–	–	–	–	–	–	–	–	–	–	–	–	–	–	–	–	–	–	
Serbia	2012	No.	137	89	0	2	3	9	3	8	21	42	48	0	1	2	2	2	1	4	35	
		Rate	1.3	1.8	0.0	1.0	1.1	3.2	1.0	2.4	1.5	2.3	0.8	0.0	0.5	0.8	0.8	0.7	0.3	0.3	1.7	

DEATHS FROM DROWNING AS REPORTED TO WHO BY COUNTRIES/AREAS CONTINUED

Notes

a Data from vital registration system with coverage estimated at 70–84%. Countries without the 'a' notation have vital registration systems with coverage estimated at 85% or higher.

b Data only available for codes W65–W74

No. Number of deaths

Rate Number of deaths per 100 000 population

– Not available/applicable

COUNTRY/AREA	YEAR	MEASURE	BOTH SEXES COMBINED	MALES									FEMALES									NOTES
				ALL	< 1	1–4	5–9	10–14	15–19	20–24	25–44	45+	ALL	< 1	1–4	5–9	10–14	15–19	20–24	25–44	45+	
Seychelles	2012	No.	6	5	0	0	1	0	1	0	1	2	1	0	0	0	0	1	0	0	0	b
		Rate	–	–	–	–	–	–	–	–	–	–	–	–	–	–	–	–	–	–	–	
Singapore	2011	No.	33	25	0	2	1	1	1	1	4	15	8	0	1	0	0	0	0	1	6	a
		Rate	0.8	1.3	0.0	2.5	0.9	0.8	0.8	0.8	0.7	2.1	0.4	0.0	1.3	0.0	0.0	0.0	0.0	0.2	0.8	
Slovakia	2010	No.	175	144	1	3	2	3	9	7	41	78	31	0	4	1	0	0	0	3	23	
		Rate	2.9	4.9	3.2	2.6	1.5	2.1	4.8	3.3	4.7	8.2	1.0	0.0	3.7	0.8	0.0	0.0	0.0	0.4	2.0	
Slovenia	2010	No.	50	32	0	0	1	0	0	2	6	23	18	0	0	0	0	0	0	1	17	
		Rate	1.7	2.5	0.0	0.0	2.1	0.0	0.0	3.0	1.9	5.4	0.9	0.0	0.0	0.0	0.0	0.0	0.0	0.3	3.5	
South Africa	2010	No.	1434	1115	10	160	144	126	113	105	278	180	319	9	92	38	46	20	16	46	51	
		Rate	2.7	4.3	1.7	7.2	5.7	5.3	4.5	4.0	3.7	3.9	1.2	1.6	4.2	1.5	2.0	0.8	0.6	0.6	0.8	
Spain	2012	No.	579	447	3	9	6	1	10	14	109	295	132	2	5	2	0	1	1	24	97	
		Rate	0.9	1.5	1.2	0.9	0.5	0.1	0.9	1.1	1.4	3.1	0.4	0.8	0.5	0.2	0.0	0.1	0.1	0.3	0.9	
Sri Lanka	2006	No.	932	716	4	26	19	33	88	73	214	259	216	3	13	13	8	9	12	58	100	a
		Rate	4.7	7.2	2.1	3.6	2.2	3.9	10.2	8.0	7.1	10.0	2.2	1.6	1.9	1.6	1.0	1.1	1.3	1.9	3.5	
Suriname	2009	No.	33	26	0	2	0	2	4	3	9	6	7	0	2	1	2	0	0	2	0	
		Rate	6.2	10.0	0.0	9.9	0.0	7.9	18.0	12.8	11.4	10.1	2.5	0.0	10.4	3.9	8.1	0.0	0.0	2.7	0.0	
Sweden	2012	No.	175	126	0	1	2	1	0	7	25	90	49	0	0	1	0	0	0	10	38	
		Rate	1.4	2.0	0.0	0.4	0.7	0.4	0.0	2.1	2.0	4.4	0.8	0.0	0.0	0.4	0.0	0.0	0.0	0.8	1.7	
Switzerland	2010	No.	102	69	0	3	0	0	5	2	14	45	33	0	0	0	0	1	0	4	28	
		Rate	1.0	1.4	0.0	1.9	0.0	0.0	2.1	0.8	1.2	2.7	0.5	0.0	0.0	0.0	0.0	0.4	0.0	0.4	1.5	
Thailand	2006	No.	4684	3578	5	358	447	175	170	164	1113	1146	1106	7	151	194	145	45	28	161	374	a
		Rate	7.3	11.2	1.2	19.6	18.0	6.7	6.4	6.2	10.6	12.5	3.6	1.7	8.7	8.2	5.8	1.8	1.1	1.5	3.6	
The former Yugoslav Republic of Macedonia	2010	No.	37	24	0	0	1	1	5	0	2	15	13	0	1	0	0	0	0	1	11	
		Rate	1.5	2.1	0.0	0.0	1.6	1.5	6.2	0.0	0.6	4.0	0.9	0.0	2.2	0.0	0.0	0.0	0.0	0.3	2.7	
Trinidad and Tobago	2008	No.	54	44	1	2	2	0	6	5	18	10	10	0	3	0	1	0	2	1	3	
		Rate	4.1	6.5	9.8	5.2	4.5	0.0	10.8	7.6	9.0	5.3	1.6	0.0	8.1	0.0	2.2	0.0	3.1	0.5	1.4	

DEATHS FROM DROWNING AS REPORTED TO WHO BY COUNTRIES/AREAS CONTINUED

Notes

a Data from vital registration system with coverage estimated at 70–84%. Countries without the 'a' notation have vital registration systems with coverage estimated at 85% or higher.

b Data only available for codes W65–W74

No. Number of deaths
Rate Number of deaths per 100 000 population
– Not available/applicable

COUNTRY/ AREA	YEAR	MEASURE	BOTH SEXES COMBINED	MALES									FEMALES									NOTES
				ALL	< 1	1–4	5–9	10–14	15–19	20–24	25–44	45+	ALL	< 1	1–4	5–9	10–14	15–19	20–24	25–44	45+	
Turkey	2011	No.	187	155	1	16	16	22	33	16	30	21	32	1	11	3	2	2	1	4	8	a
		Rate	0.3	0.4	0.2	0.6	0.5	0.7	1.0	0.5	0.3	0.2	0.1	0.2	0.5	0.1	0.1	0.1	0.0	0.0	0.1	
Turks and Caicos Islands	2009	No.	18	2	0	0	0	0	1	0	0	1	16	0	0	0	0	0	0	0	16	
		Rate	–	–	–	–	–	–	–	–	–	–	–	–	–	–	–	–	–	–	–	
Ukraine	2012	No.	2713	2303	2	38	50	30	86	159	824	1113	410	2	18	13	26	23	11	93	224	b
		Rate	5.5	9.8	0.8	3.7	4.6	3.0	6.8	9.4	12.1	14.2	1.6	0.8	1.9	1.3	2.7	1.9	0.7	1.4	1.9	
United Kingdom	2010	No.	578	437	3	8	4	6	25	34	112	245	141	0	4	0	3	1	7	32	94	
		Rate	0.8	1.2	0.7	0.5	0.2	0.3	1.2	1.5	1.3	2.0	0.4	0.0	0.3	0.0	0.2	0.1	0.3	0.4	0.7	
United States of America	2010	No.	4812	3687	34	311	106	97	297	366	979	1495	1125	25	159	37	27	33	61	233	550	
		Rate	1.5	2.4	1.6	3.7	1.0	0.9	2.6	3.3	2.3	2.6	0.7	1.3	2.0	0.4	0.3	0.3	0.6	0.6	0.8	
Uruguay	2010	No.	137	101	0	2	2	4	18	9	21	44	36	0	2	2	2	4	0	6	20	
		Rate	3.9	6.0	0.0	2.0	1.6	3.0	13.4	7.2	4.7	8.4	1.9	0.0	2.1	1.6	1.6	3.1	0.0	1.3	3.0	
Uzbekistan	2005	No.	1053	710	0	214	74	56	39	35	188	104	343	4	182	35	37	14	13	37	21	a
		Rate	4.0	5.6	0.0	20.4	5.1	3.4	2.5	2.7	5.1	5.0	2.5	1.6	18.4	2.5	2.3	0.9	1.0	1.0	0.9	
Venezuela (Bolivarian Republic of)	2009	No.	645	539	11	68	32	27	94	81	154	72	106	7	40	17	12	10	4	9	7	
		Rate	2.1	3.6	3.6	5.7	2.2	1.9	6.8	6.0	3.7	2.3	0.7	2.4	3.5	1.2	0.9	0.7	0.3	0.2	0.2	
Virgin Islands (USA)	2010	No.	4	2	0	0	0	0	1	0	0	1	2	0	0	0	0	0	0	0	2	
		Rate	–	–	–	–	–	–	–	–	–	–	–	–	–	–	–	–	–	–	–	

Photography credits

Cover: Getty Images/iStock/D. Freund Photography
Page ii: WHO/A. Kari
Page vi: Getty Images/iStock/Gremlin
Page viii: Getty Images/iStock/B. Hadyniak
Page x: Getty Images/iStock/Skynavin
Page 2: Getty Images/iStock/Peeterv
Page 4: Getty Images/iStock/G. Delmotte Photography
Page 8: WHO/SEARO/R. Kumar
Page 11: Getty Images/iStock/Mathess
Page 13: Getty Images/Stockbyte
Page 14: Getty Images/iStock/PeskyMonkey
Page 16: Getty Images/iStock/Enviromantic
Page 17: Jonathan Guevarra
Page 20: Getty Images/iStock/M&H Sheppard
Page 21: Getty Images/iStock/EPSTOCK
Page 23: WHO/WPRO
Page 24, top: Getty Images/iStock/Lokibaho
Page 24, bottom: Aminur Rahman
Page 27: Getty Images/iStock/Motionteam Photo Press
Page 29: Getty Images/iStock/D. Freund Photography
Page 31: Getty Images/iStock/Meinzahn
Page 32: Getty Images/iStock/Turhanyalcin
Page 34: Getty Images/iStock/Ruchos
Page 35: Getty Images/iStock/B. Hadyniak
Page 37: Getty Images/iStock/Hottest Tea
Page 38: Getty Images/Moment Open/Shibu Bhattacharjee
Page 40: Getty Images/iStock/Tina Baxter
Inside Cover: Getty Images/Moment Open/Yasir Arafat

Design and graphics

AHOY Studios, ahoystudios.com

Made possible by funding from

Bloomberg Philanthropies